'As warm and entertai...   ...humour
shines through the tri...   ...vet.'
...Leonard

'A great little book that will make both tails and tongues wag.'
David Bellamy

'Right from the Introduction any animal lover will be drawn
into this enchanting and amusing account of veterinary life.
Emma Milne tells of her early career as a vet in practice,
in a brilliantly honest and warm way, vividly recounting
the ups and downs of the novice vet. A highly entertaining
read coupled with the obvious passion that Emma has for
her subject matter. James Herriot, in his country practice,
would have much in common with this version of life as an
animals' doctor.'
Clarissa Baldwin OBE

'Emma is a classic twenty-first-century vet; young, female and
opinionated, with reality-television celebrity status. Her tales
– of animals, farmers, pet owners and television cameras – are
both engaging and entertaining.'
Pete Wedderburn, the *Daily Telegraph* vet

'A bluntly honest and eye-opening book that takes one on
a most fascinating journey behind the traditional "shop
front" of the veterinary world... an absolute must-read for
all animal lovers.'
Allen Parton, author of *Endal*

'*Funny and pertinent to all of us who have pets, and probably disturbing for those that don't!*' Rick Wakeman

'*This book is delightful, amusing and honest, like Emma.*' Christopher Timothy

'*A sensitive but sometimes harrowing account of the challenges facing a greenhorn vet directly out of vet school. I found this book a joy to read. I could relate to the fears and exhilaration that Emma felt in those early days and how her confidence gained momentum. The learning curve will continue through her life, but with Emma at the helm, it could only be good for our animal friends.*' Terry Nutkins

'*I have every respect for someone who can put their hand up a half-ton cow, and then pull it out to write so engagingly about the experience.*' Andrew Dilger, author of *Dash: Bitch of the Year*

'*Like reading a transcript of my first job,* Tales from the Tail End *captures a vet's journey from student to practicing clinician brilliantly... with liberal yet totally well-founded splatterings of crazy when describing our beloved clients and ourselves. A great read!*' Scott Miller

Tales from the
TAIL END

Adventures of a
Vet in Practice

Emma Milne

with a foreword by Brian Blessed

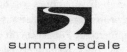

summersdale

TALES FROM THE TAIL END

Copyright © Emma Milne, 2012

All rights reserved.

No part of this book may be reproduced by any means, nor transmitted, nor translated into a machine language, without the written permission of the publishers.

The right of Emma Milne to be identified as the author of this work has been asserted in accordance with sections 77 and 78 of the Copyright, Designs and Patents Act 1988.

Condition of Sale
This book is sold subject to the condition that it shall not, by way of trade or otherwise, be lent, re-sold, hired out or otherwise circulated in any form of binding or cover other than that in which it is published and without a similar condition including this condition being imposed on the subsequent publisher.

Summersdale Publishers Ltd
46 West Street
Chichester
West Sussex
PO19 1RP
UK

www.summersdale.com

Printed and bound in Great Britain

ISBN: 978-1-84953-213-6

Substantial discounts on bulk quantities of Summersdale books are available to corporations, professional associations and other organisations. For details telephone Summersdale Publishers on (+44-1243-771107), fax (+44-1243-786300) or email (nicky@summersdale.com).

For Mum and Dad for teaching me that childhoods full of laughter, love and happiness are the richest there are.

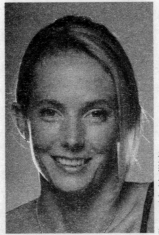
Photograph by John Wright

About the author

Emma Milne qualified from Bristol Vet School in 1996 and was featured in all eleven series of the BBC television programme *Vets in Practice*. Since qualifying, Emma has been a general veterinary practitioner, and she has also worked in television and media and written for many publications. Her passion for animal welfare has led her to become involved with several charities, and she is also a patron of Dogs Trust and a trustee of the BVA Animal Welfare Foundation. In 2008 she received the International Fund for Animal Welfare Vet of the Year award for highlighting their work in the townships of South Africa.

You can read more about Emma at her website, **www.emmathevet.co.uk**, and follow her on Twitter, **@EmmaMilneTheVet**.

Contents

Foreword by Brian Blessed..9

Introduction...11

Chapter 1
About as much use as a kick in the... 13

Chapter 2
Whatever the weather..33

Chapter 3
This is a man's world, but it wouldn't be nothin'... 58

Chapter 4
To sleep, perchance to dream..................................78

Chapter 5
Mirror, mirror, on the wall... 102

Chapter 6
Brian strikes again...119

Chapter 7
Stick it to me..138

Chapter 8
Till Death Us Do Part..157

Chapter 9
There's now't as queer as folk...............................179

Chapter 10
What goes in doesn't always come out....................199

Chapter 11
It really shouldn't happen to a vet..........................223

Afterword...250

Foreword

by Brian Blessed

Reading this book has proved to be a delightful, stunning experience. It is a celebration, an account of some of the adventures in the early life of a young vet. I simply couldn't put it down! Emma Milne writes with gravitas and soul, combined with a rare gift for infectious humour. You must forgive me if I sound too exuberant. I must confess that I am totally biased towards the whole veterinary profession!

The other day I had the task of pushing a chubby Shetland pony out of the kitchen as it devoured the dog food and filled the floor with a good supply of manure. For the past 45 years everything I have earned has gone on protecting our livestock. Scores of different farmyard ducks: Aylesburies, Khaki Campbells, Muscovies, black Cayugas, raucous Call Ducks plus dozens of hens, not to mention numerous ponies and dogs and cats and birds of the air who eat us out of house and home, a veritable 'Noah's Ark' made possible by the love, energy and care of our vets. In all weathers they turn up and perform minor miracles. It is often said by the discerning that qualifying to be a vet is a harder test than becoming a GP. They have my unstinting admiration.

This book is a tour de force – Emma is such a terrific writer. *Vets in Practice* was a wonderful TV series. I never missed an episode.

Boys and girls, ladies and gentlemen, I urge you to immerse yourself in this book and emerge at the end with every cell in your body happily changed!

Introduction

The recipe for a vet's life:

1. Take a mix of people who are sad, happy, angry and sometimes plainly barking mad. Take a few years to realise that these are just your colleagues.
2. Add a heaped bucketful of clients who are altogether madder, sadder and badder (and hopefully some happy ones too).
3. Stir in an equal number of their animals, ranging from pot-bellied pigs to hamsters.
4. Add a hearty spoonful of the animals' attitudes, ranging from enthusiastic slobbering to a low warning snarl to a hefty kick in the nether regions.
5. Simmer with expectation throughout childhood and allow to boil over uncontrollably once qualified.
6. To add the topping and make it my life, add a film crew for seven years, a working life in the media spotlight and a personal life exposed for all to see.

OR:

Simply sit back, relax and revel in someone else's misfortune.

You may have seen some of the antics in these pages on television, you might have read snippets in magazines over the years, but now I've got the chance to let you into the whole unadulterated and often messy affair in all its glory. Many of the names have been changed, purely to protect the heinously guilty. I hope you enjoy it as much as I did!

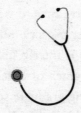

Chapter 1

About as much use as a kick in the...

The kick hit me square in the pelvis. I didn't even have time to flinch because I didn't see it coming. My head was turned and I was talking to the farmer. Even if my brain had noticed the lightning-fast flash of white in my peripheral vision it would have barely made it out of its armchair and picked up its loudhailer to yell at my legs to move me out of the way before, a split second later, the cloven hoof of half a ton of disgruntled dairy cow connected with my bladder and launched me about two metres backwards. Standing, as I had been, about a metre away from her when she cast a malevolent eye over her shoulder to take aim is about as bad a place as you can be when a cow decides she didn't actually appreciate the much-talked-about hand up her backside. If you want to avoid being injured by horses and cows, you should make sure you are either well out of a surprisingly long striking distance or pressed closely against the back end. The latter may seem insane but the point is that the kick doesn't have time to wind up to its full, lethal potential and you just get a gentle nudge. Standing midway between these two places is utterly stupid and I should think the black-and-white daughter of Satan couldn't believe her luck when this fresh young graduate so kindly parked herself there and then *looked in the other direction!* I wouldn't have minded but I'd finished what I was doing, and the whole time I was actually furtling around in her insides she hadn't batted an eyelid. All the better to lull me in for the sucker punch, I suppose. I bet there was much hilarity and bovine guffawing over the food trough that night.

As I landed, doubled over like a human pair of kitchen tongs, I realised with a detached interest that I'd let out a primeval guttural yell without even realising it. I think it was the caveman-esque scream combined with the distance I moved not of my own free will, which had left the farmer looking ashen and open-mouthed, like a slightly stunned goldfish. I raised my head to look at him as I clutched my abdomen and, after what seemed like a very long time, he finally managed to whisper, 'Are you OK?' At this point I stood upright, mentally shook myself like a dog ridding itself of water, said, 'Yes, I'm fine,' and calmly continued what I'd been telling him about the reproductive state of his herd. I gathered my belongings, sauntered off to my car and left the farm. It wasn't until I got back to the surgery and reported what had happened to one of the two lovely ladies who brought a little sunshine into my working life and the adrenalin stopped flowing that I crumpled into a pathetic girly mess and started bawling my eyes out.

Having rung the local doctor and been told to 'keep an eye out and if you start bleeding into your urine, let me know', I started to get the inkling that, after only a month in the job, maybe being a vet wasn't going to be a bed of roses after all. As I would soon discover, this was to be one of a string of many weird and wonderful things which would happen to me over the years since starting vet school. So many of us, having devotedly watched James Herriot through our formative years, thought, 'Yes, actually I *would* like to spend my life with my arm up a cow's bum.' Being one of them, I strove with all my brainpower and any charm I could muster to persuade the people on the interview panels that their vet school would be so much better with me in it. But, as you'll see, life as a vet is not as straightforward, warm or fuzzy as you may have been led to believe.

I thought I'd tackle the whole cow's bum thing right from the get-go because on behalf of the profession I'd like to put it to bed here and now. From the second you make the decision, if you tell anyone you want to be a vet they will invariably within thirty seconds or so say, 'Oh, you must want to spend your life with your hand up a cow's bum.' Strange as it may seem, there *is* slightly more to the five-year course and the lifetime of work but, as I always say on the subject of cows' bums, you won't find many warmer places to keep your hands on a farm in the middle of winter.

Having spent my five years at vet school in the warm haze of a sheltered and coddled existence, helped along by brilliant teachers, a few tyrants and quite a lot of booze, the reality of being thrust into the outside world hit me like the rounders bat I once got in the way of in primary school. I was hugely in debt and the bank and the government thought it was high time I knuckled down, stopped sponging off the taxpayers and started actually paying my way in society. Along with the prospect of a lifetime spent chipping away at my credit mountain, I also found myself positively bursting with knowledge, and desperate to start saving lives and cutting into people's animals, preferably with their permission and for a genuine reason! Now all I needed was a job.

There is a weekly publication called the *Veterinary Record*, where accomplished vets with more letters after their names than friends (yes, jealousy is an ugly thing!) like to get their research published. Most of the articles are so scientific and densely packed with charts, graphs and very long words that to the mere mortals of the veterinary world they are indecipherable, but the *Record* is also the place to go to find a job. The vacant positions are found towards the back, and, along with the obituaries, are the most thumbed pages of the publication. One of the brilliant things about being a vet is that you can take the work wherever you want to go. I had no mortgage, no kids and the whole world was at my feet. But I *did* have a boyfriend and said boyfriend liked to surf and had already got a job in Bideford in Devon. The world receded to a small corner of the country unless I wanted to jettison the boyfriend, but I liked him a lot and so I started scouring the south-west for a job. I found *one* that was close enough to be reasonable. So my little world suddenly became a dot on the edge of Exmoor called Dulverton.

Dulverton is a picture-postcard village and the practice that had saved my relationship was offering what we call 'a very mixed job'. This means a practice which caters for the needs of large and small animals alike and, in their case, this probably erred very slightly on the side of farm work. I was looking for a mixed job, like many new graduates, because I hadn't decided yet what I'd like to specialise in and wanted to get a good all-round taster of what it was all about.

The basic salary was pretty low, but with accommodation provided and good money towards a car on top, the whole package was enough to make a totally skint former student's eyes pop out and conjure up images of a grand lifestyle. As I hastily accepted the job for fear it would vanish before my eyes, I reluctantly had to admit to myself that it was time to say goodbye to my good friend Billy.

I loved Billy dearly and he had been with me through thick and thin during my last two years at university. He had stoically taken everything I had burdened him with, had never minded my moods and had always done his best to help me get to where I needed to be in life. But the sad truth was that my clapped-out, faithful little black Mini just wasn't up to farm work on Exmoor. I could have piled the equipment in the back seat, as I had with my worldly possessions in between term times for the trek back and forth between Kent and Bristol, but the fact was that navigating the shallowest of puddles now caused an inevitable flooding of the gubbins under the bonnet followed by immediate engine failure. Throughout the holidays from university he'd loyally taken me all over the country 'seeing practice'. This is what all vet students have to do and simply means we get to shadow (or intensely annoy) 'real' vets at their places of work. It gives students a good idea of the day-to-day business of vetting and also allows for extra hands-on experience before being unleashed into the real world. For the last few months of seeing practice I had had to hang out of Billy's door and 'skateboard' him down the hill outside my parents' house to get enough momentum to bump-start him every day. He had to go.

My dad said he'd take him as a runabout so at least I knew he would be in safe hands with the family. I agreed on the strict understanding that my pesky sister Alice, seven years my junior and just learning to drive, was under no circumstances to get her thieving and irresponsible young hands on him. I must have been out of the house for about thirty seconds before he was handed over to the toerag. I suppose I shouldn't have been surprised. When I left to go to uni in the first place I was told solemnly that 'your bedroom will always be there for you. It will always be yours as long as you want it.' The first weekend I came home I found that Alice had bloody moved into it from the room she 'cosily' shared with our youngest sister, Rebecca, and I was now relegated to the bed-settee in the lounge. I was starting to realise that it's true what they say: families – you can't live with 'em, you can't kill 'em!

I arrived in the village of Dulverton in 1996 as a wide-eyed twenty-four-year-old with my few possessions in a shiny new second-hand car. I was very vocally joined on my journey by my three-legged cat Charlie, who had found his way into my life while I was doing a few weeks' locum work after qualifying. The house that came with the job was down a small row, which ran along an alley perpendicular to the main road. I had to double-park to get anywhere near the place and was worried about being arrested and carted off before I managed to start work. I stopped a woman in the street and asked her if she thought it would be OK to park there while I unloaded a few things. Her immediate reply was, 'Oh, you must be the new vet then.' I flicked my eyes from one side to the other in a rather fearful glance for some clue as to how this total stranger knew who I was and, finding nothing, managed a weak smile and confirmed her suspicions. It seemed that Dulverton was going to be one of those places where people knew your business before you did.

Mum and Dad were planning to stay the weekend to help me find my feet in the village and celebrate the move, but the celebrations were quickly put on hold when we discovered to our horror that Charlie had legged it (or limped it) into foreign and unknown territory. I had visions of my poor disabled half-grown kitten sheltering alone in the damp recesses of this strange new place, and of me never being able to find him. After a family search party, which included a lot of tin-can-banging and name-calling, and the enlisting of several very helpful and eager villagers, we had to admit defeat. We went home depressed and sat in a draughty house with the front door open in the hope that he would somehow find his way back.

After what seemed like hours I was sure I had heard his very distinct and plaintive meow. I told everyone to be quiet. We all strained to listen and after a few minutes there it was again. We were sure of it now but where was he? I walked slowly and painstakingly round the house, pausing until I heard the next sound, until I finally narrowed it down to a bedroom upstairs. There I found a terrified and hungry scrap of a cat wedged behind one of the wardrobes. He hadn't even left the house. My relief was unbounded and the mood lightened considerably for the rest of the evening as my parents were finally able to help me unpack. Thankfully, Charlie didn't seem any the worse for his adventure. Before long, this beautiful little three-quarter cat grew to be a formidable presence in the village and ruled the roost wherever he went.

Inevitably, come Sunday afternoon, my parents had to leave to wend their way back to Kent, navigating the big car park best known as the M25. So it was that I found myself all alone, apart from a slightly aloof, biscuit-coloured, former stray who thought life was just a big ball of wool to chase. Reality slowly dawned on me. Tomorrow was the first day of my fledgling career and I really would be on my own.

Monday morning finally came after a long and sleepless night and I got ready for work with a sense of utterly debilitating fear. It suddenly seemed to me that every fact I had ever learnt at university had somehow, in the few weeks between qualifying and landing in Exmoor, vanished without a trace from my brain. All I could think about was a vet called Paul, with whom I used to see practice in the holidays, who had told me about the five stages of knowledge. Ironically, I couldn't remember the details of that either but I did remember the gist and that the first stage is that new graduates know so little that they don't even know they don't know anything. On that dank and grey Monday morning I had no illusions on this score and wanted to run for the hills, screaming, and find somewhere to hide. From nine o'clock that morning people were going to bring their animals to me and expect me to know what was wrong with them. I wasn't the student standing in the corner anymore. The buck stopped with me and I was, for want of a better expression, bricking it!

From the day of my job interview I recalled that the surgery was what could be described as quaint, or even ramshackle, but it had a kind of antiquated charm. Where most modern surgeries are made of miles of gleaming chrome, most of the fixtures and fittings here were wooden. The building was small with a tiny consulting room, a small operating theatre upstairs and what can only be described as a cupboard for taking X-rays in. This was one of many surgeries doing mainly large-animal work, and which therefore had no need for large or flashy premises or acres of sophisticated equipment, because so much farm work is done out of the boot of your car. Upstairs there were a couple of gas heaters as the only source of warmth and, most intriguingly, shelf upon shelf of various sizes of brown glass bottles with big stoppers in them. Having come from a state-of-the-art university, I felt like I'd gone back in time by about a century. It turned out the bottles contained an assortment of weird and wonderful lotions and potions, home-made remedies which had been made and passed down through generations. For all I knew, some of them still had the original potions *in* them. Discovering that one of them had ether in it didn't make me any less nervous, considering that the senior partner, Mr Elliot, used to chain-smoke while wandering among the cramped and highly explosive collection.

Mr Elliot had terrified me from the moment I arrived for my interview. I had always been a bit timid in certain circumstances but in hindsight I wish I had then been more who I am today because I think I would have found him a different being altogether. He's one of the most memorable people I've ever met and he also had one of the most incredible memories I've ever encountered. I've since realised after years in the job myself that, if you repeat the same things every day, as vets do, you eventually get ingrained knowledge that is difficult to shed. At the time, however, I was simply in awe of the breadth of information he held in his brain.

Every single vet I've known or worked with over the years has been referred to by their first name, except Mr Elliot. The first time a farmer said that 'Don' had been out the week before me I had no idea who he was talking about. It took a few moments of gormless staring while the cogs clattered round in my head to realise, not only that my boss *had* a first name and that it was Don, but that some people were actually allowed to call him that.

Mr Elliot was a small, wiry man with the complexion of someone who's had nicotine loitering round their skin for decades. He often scowled but equally often let out bellowing laughter at one of his own jokes. There seemed to be nothing in between these two moods. He would look like thunder if anyone dared to ring up for a visit. When Bretia or Mary, the two wonderful ladies who covered every job from nurse to cleaner to receptionist, leaned away from the phone to tell him who wanted to speak to him, he would exhale a string of expletives at the top of his voice about whoever was on the other end of the phone and there was no doubt that the poor farmer could hear every word of it. The mouthpiece would be hastily covered just a few seconds too late and after a great deal of huffing and puffing he'd snatch the phone and have a totally normal conversation, fixing the problem there and then with advice, or genially agreeing to be there at his own convenience, before hanging up and continuing the huffing and swearing. Without a shadow of a doubt, Mr Elliot swore more than any other person I've ever known. I was in no doubt that working alongside this enigma of a man would be what my mum would call 'character building'!

Long before I qualified, at the start of my final year at university, the BBC in Bristol had come up with the novel idea of making a programme about final-year vet students and, having come to meet our motley crew, they decided we had enough oddballs and characters in our year to make it worthwhile. The filming of *Vets School* induced mixed feelings among the staff and students. Some of us thought it was very exciting to have the film crews lurking about the place while others were filled with horror at the impact that canny editing might have on the reputations of all concerned. The six-part series went out without a single hint of myself in it, apart from a fleeting glimpse of my rather shabby shoes in an RSPCA clinic where

I was on placement. My shoes wouldn't have been in it either had it not been for the fact that Alison, who was being featured, ended up examining a rabbit that I'd been filmed with first and they needed some footage of the hapless, paralyzed creature at the time of its first consultation with me.

I'd be lying if I said I wasn't a little disappointed at having been guillotined mercilessly from the production, especially when it turned out that the public bloody loved it. As it transpired, though, all was not lost and the viewing figures prompted those wise men at the Beeb to commission the follow-up series *Vets in Practice*. That summer I had received a phone call asking if I'd be happy to be featured in the new series (as had my boyfriend, Joe), and I had jumped at the chance and rung my prospective bosses in Dulverton to get the go-ahead from them. With green lights all round, I thought I was definitely 'ready for my close-up' now.

And so it was on that Monday morning that, added to my fear about having to know how to treat sick animals, I realised with startling clarity that, instead of fame and fortune, what was probably about to happen was that the BBC were going to highlight my thickest and most embarrassing moments for the foreseeable future. Right on time, an hour before I was due to wander the hundred metres from home to work, a crew of four arrived at the house to capture the look of terror on my young, spotty face. As it turned out, starting work and being responsible for animals' lives was so incredibly terrifying that I hardly noticed the camera crew.

I arrived at work with my little entourage and was very relieved to see that I hadn't been put on the rota for morning surgery. This relief was quickly squashed when Mr Elliot strode in to the room, managed a disgusted grunt by way of welcoming the BBC to his humble practice, and told me my first job was to go on a farm visit to a goat with a bad eye. Oh Christ. My shrivelled brain started frantically scouring itself for information about goats' eye diseases. When it came up empty it tried goats and then eyes separately and still came up blank. It shrugged its shoulders, settled back down into its armchair and said, 'Sorry, kid, but you're on your own.' This internal monologue had clearly left my face either contorted with horror or totally blank and gormless, because the all-knowing wizard that was Mr Elliot grabbed a box of small tubes of ointment from the shelf, thrust one at me and said, 'Just make sure there's nothing stuck in it and give them this to use for five days.'

The farm in question turned out to have a bit of a mixture of animals. A large barn and meadow were there for free-range egg production, which was the mainstay of the farm's income, but as the owner, Jan, showed me round, more and more animals of various shapes and sizes appeared, from sheep and lambs to ponies to a voluminous Vietnamese pot-bellied pig. Jan was the kind of woman you immediately warmed to. She had an open, happy face, and very quickly put me at ease. It's very difficult as a brand new graduate to have faith in your own abilities but she left me in no doubt that she, surprisingly, *did* have total trust in me. After our brief tour of the beautifully kept place I had a strong feeling not only that she was a wonderful owner and keeper of animals, someone who really cared, but also that we might become good friends given half a chance.

By the time I got to the goat I was feeling like I had been welcomed to my new position as vet and, being a little more relaxed, recalled what all vets do instinctively when presented with any animal, which is start from scratch. People are always commenting to vets that it must be much harder for us than doctors because animals can't tell us what's wrong, but I've always viewed this differently, because it is for that very reason that we always try to get a thorough history and carry out a full examination of the whole animal. We probably don't get bogged down as doctors may do by people banging on about one problem when there is really something else going on. A bad eye may well just be a bad eye but it can also be a sign of a much deeper disease, which an owner may not know about. I also realised quite quickly as a recent graduate that doing a full clinical exam also gives you time to think! In fact the goat was very well and in great condition apart from a red and infected eye. As Mr Elliot had predicted I handed over the tube of antibiotic ointment, labelled with instructions, and gave my first official farm-animal diagnosis and advice. It felt great!

A couple of hours after I'd left the surgery I triumphantly returned, reputation as yet unscathed, having treated a goat with conjunctivitis. I had actually found once I got started that I did in fact know some veterinary medicine. Maybe this wasn't going to be as hard as I imagined.

Or at least that's what I thought until about ten o'clock that night, which turned out to be the first night I was on call. This came as a bit of a shock but since my predecessor's departure Mr Elliot and the other partner, Martin, had been handling the already fairly savage rota on their own, and I suppose they must have been overjoyed to have just about anyone to help, even a wet-behind-the-ears new graduate. For everything that was spiky about Mr Elliot, there was the opposite in Martin. He was a wonderfully gentle and incredibly quiet man who seemed to exude tranquillity. I wondered in those early days how they managed to get along but I suspect that, just as opposite poles attract, they actually complemented each other perfectly.

The phone call came as I was contemplating bed after what had been in truth a pretty easy day, but after all the tension, coupled with the nerves and the film crew, I was exhausted. The tone of the woman's voice on the phone left no doubt that I wasn't going to bed and the adrenalin started pumping the life back in to me. Their dog had collapsed and was unresponsive: they desperately needed help. I said I'd meet them at the surgery as soon as they could get there.

As agreed, I rang the film crew to tell them there was an emergency coming down and I headed the mercifully short distance back to work. After about twenty minutes a car pulled into the car park and a middle-aged couple carried a totally recumbent and barely-conscious Border collie called Beth into the surgery. We laid her on the consulting room table and I did a quick check on her vital signs. Her breath was shallow and rapid, her heart was racing and her gums were as white as a sheet. I took a blood sample and ran upstairs to get the sample running and get the makings of a drip to start treating her dangerously collapsed state.

There was, almost immediately, an urgent shout from the sound man in the film crew and I dashed back downstairs.

Every face in the room told the same story and then someone said, 'She just stopped breathing'. The dog was, to all intents and purposes, dead on the table. Automatic pilot kicked in and I started CPR. After thirty seconds or so she took a shuddering breath and her heart started again. We carried her between us up the awkward stairs and into the operating theatre, where there was all the equipment we might need. As soon as she was on oxygen I leapt for the phone, knowing I was well and truly out of my depth. Martin's wife, an equally tranquil vet who was expecting twins so had drastically reduced her hours at the practice, soon arrived, ousted the disappointed film crew and we got to work on the dog. A quickly placed needle and syringe into the abdomen came back full of blood – a dire sign. We got a drip of blood replacement fluids started and gave medication for shock but the dog was so weak that exploratory surgery was out of the question. All we could do was wait in the hope that the morning might bring the news that she was stronger and that the source of the bleeding had dried up and stopped.

Sadly, this was not to be and my first job the next morning was to ring Beth's doting owners and tell them that she had died from her injuries. They asked us to do a post mortem and it showed that she had a ruptured liver. The owners thought she might have been kicked by one of their ponies and that could certainly have been the cause. It is inevitable that as a vet, and often as an owner, you will ask yourself if there was anything else you could have done. As a new graduate I tortured myself about this for many nights. I was so proud that I'd managed to bring her back with CPR, but in all likelihood her blood loss was so great and she was so desperately ill by the time I saw her that nothing and no one could have saved her. It is human nature to wonder, though. What if we'd had the staff and facilities of a university? But the fact remains that we didn't, and one of the hardest things to come to terms with as a vet is not being able to save an animal. We have such incredible medicine, technology and knowledge now that it is easy to feel invincible, especially in a university setting. But the harsh reality in the real world is that money, time and circumstances are by no means always on your side and this was a lesson it seemed I was fated to start learning from day one.

My first twenty-four hours were certainly eventful but in many ways that was for the best. I'd had to cope on my own with a number of situations and start to snip away at the apron strings of my university days but this had also shown me that, whatever the surgery lacked in fancy equipment, they made up for with brilliant vets and fantastic support out of hours, which for a new graduate is priceless. When I was seeing practice a vet had once said to me, when I was panicking about being unleashed into general practice, 'Concentrate on getting through your first day, then your first week, and you won't believe how quickly it all starts to become second nature.' It seemed impossible to believe after *my* first day but by Friday that week I could see what he meant. I was starting to get into the flow of things. Every day was a learning experience but every day brought a little more confidence and I was loving the job. All that remained was for me to get through my last afternoon surgery of the week and then I had the weekend off so I could relax for a couple of days.

The practice had an open surgery policy, which meant that clients could turn up any time during the half-hour slots given over to the surgeries. On paper these looked like brilliantly short and easy sessions to deal with, but in reality people would lounge around at home leaving you twiddling your thumbs for twenty-nine minutes then arrive en masse and keep you there for two hours, making you late for all your farm visits.

Unbeknown to me, this particular afternoon was going to bring the first of many lessons to come about client-vet relationships. It is a classic mistake that many young people make when deciding they want to be a vet that they want to do so because they want to work with animals. Yes, you do work with animals, but 99.9 per cent of those animals are going to come to you with a person attached. Some will be wonderful, some will be awful, some will be distraught and some will be stark raving mad, but deal with them you must. What I was about to find out was that many people seem to view vets as being somewhere between a priest and a doctor. We are bound by the confidentiality of the consulting room confessional and there is a long-perpetuated myth that being a vet is harder than being a doctor so therefore we must be better or more intelligent somehow. In truth this myth is largely perpetuated by vets, because it makes us feel smug and superior to doctors when actually we're just jealous of their salaries and on-call hours.

I wasn't feeling too stressed about afternoon surgery because I'd gained a lot more practical experience with small-animal medicine and surgery than with farm animals over my years of studying. I'd seen a couple of clients, nothing taxing so far, when a middle-aged woman arrived with a small, enthusiastic spaniel. The woman had gone past 'rounded', sailed straight through 'sturdy' and had arrived at 'chunky' – and she was showing no signs of going back. The eager little spaniel leapt nimbly onto the table as the woman started to explain that she wasn't really worried about the dog but she just wanted to know what the creatures crawling all over it were.

I leaned in to take a closer look because at first glance I couldn't actually see anything on the dog at all. My eyes adjusted to the coat colour and I realised that, brilliantly camouflaged, there was a veritable army of small ticks. I'd never in my life seen so many. Most ticks we see are the big obvious ones, which are fat, grey, full to bursting with blood and on their own, often mistaken for small growths or warts by unsuspecting owners. The critters which had hitched a ride on this little spaniel were just babies and they hadn't yet had time to burrow through the fur to their mission's target of the skin and the gorgeous, warm blood vessels that reside there.

I mentally sat on my hands to resist the urge to start frantically scratching and told the owner what they were. In fact she was to be commended for spotting the tiny creatures so early and bringing the dog in. I explained that with a quick application of a recently launched wonder spray the dog would be parasite-free and back on the moors, wedged happily, nose down and bottom up, into the undergrowth looking for mischief. I'd just started to write the notes when the woman, without batting an eyelid or skipping a beat, said, 'Oh, do you think that might be what *this* is?' and, with great speed and an unabashed flourish that would have made a lap dancer proud, she whipped off her whole blouse, revealing an expanse of squidgy, blotchy flesh and lifted one arm. Too late I tried, and failed, to avert my eyes from her ample bosom, light-pink silky bra and neatly shaved armpit. Nestled in that same pristine armpit was the unmistakable, shiny, plump form of a very happy, very large and very adult tick. I froze in horror on so many different levels and tried to find my voice. Eventually I composed myself, raised my eyebrows and said simply, 'Yes, it is,' and then advised her it would be best to show it to her doctor, who presumably was fully equipped mentally and physically to deal with both the parasite and the expanse of flesh in which it was lodged.

Having dispatched the now fully dressed woman, her new best friend and her parasite-ridden charge to the waiting room, I wrote the label for the spray and made a mental note to myself to get a chair for the consulting room. If this was going to happen regularly I was really going to need somewhere to sit down.

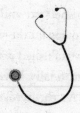

Chapter 2

Whatever the weather

It seemed that those first few weeks flew by. The practice was very busy and as I'd started in October the winter descended oh-so-quickly; I soon discovered some home truths about doing farm animal work on the moors all year round. Come to think about it, I soon discovered that the lovely little house that came with the job was also just an extension of the outside masquerading as a house.

It was nestled in a small terraced row built of typical Exmoor stone and seemed to shimmer in that damp way that only English houses can. There were two bedrooms upstairs and a living-room-cum-diner downstairs leading to a kitchen. Tucked downstairs was also the bathroom, which had a high ceiling and a huge skylight making it, on first appearances, a lovely light space with a big luxurious bath. There was an open fire in the living room which, over the years, has become a priority of mine in a house, simply because I have always been mesmerised by naked flames. I think this is a primeval instinct that mankind hasn't quite shed yet and I love to sit by the fire listening to the crackle and spit of the wood.

When I first moved in I was flushed with excitement about the job, the house, the car and finally having achieved my dream of saving animals' lives. As the weeks trundled by and the temperature gradually dropped, I finally noticed that the only source of heat in the house besides the fire were two small storage heaters – one downstairs and one upstairs. Anyone who's lived in a house reliant on this form of heating anywhere outside the equatorial region will no doubt know what a totally useless way to heat a house it is. All the heaters accomplished was stopping the temperature in the house actually reaching zero. It soon became apparent that I was going to need multiple trips to the little supermarket a few doors away for logs and coal and, sure enough, my puny arms started to grow the muscles that I'd need when it came to wrestling beef cattle onto the ground.

One of my most resounding memories of the house is sitting as close to the open fire as I could get with the fire absolutely roaring, and with my clothes, coat, hat, scarf and gloves on, and *just about* being warm enough. It was on these occasions that I was grateful for my capacious bladder – at a push, it could hold about two litres, I reckon – because I had come to regard going to the bathroom with a feeling of dread. The lovely skylight was actually the perfect conduit for ejecting heat out of the house faster than I could produce it. If I tried the age-old cold-defying remedy of having a scorching hot bath, I was then faced with the problem of trying to get out of the bath directly under the arctic portal that was the skylight and getting dressed before all the heat from the bath and indeed my soul was sucked out of my body. It became a balancing act of trying to get used to being superheated to about fifty degrees just to compensate for the heat that would be lost between exiting the water, getting dried and getting dressed again. I soon came to the conclusion that it wasn't worth all the effort and opted for huddling by the fire instead. My evenings of frantic coal-shovelling started to resemble the engine room of a steam passenger liner. I was beginning to wonder if I just wasn't cut out for life on the moors.

Forty minutes away, by the sea, Joe's cushy number in Bideford had him visiting beautifully organised dairy farms with their obligatory hot water, soap and towels, and with cows in deep straw beds in large, comfy barns. My job was more of a baptism by fire, or more correctly, ice. The farm animals we handled were very different to Joe's dairy cows. Not for me, those much-handled and docile beasts so accustomed to their human carers. Oh no, the moors favoured slightly wilder beef cattle and sheep who might catch a glimpse of a human occasionally over a hedge but certainly didn't take kindly to being touched by one. Exmoor is a very beautiful place and on crisp winter mornings when the sun was shining and the frost was layered thick on the ground you couldn't find a more lovely place to be. Unless, that is, you had to actually go outside with bits of your body exposed. Some of our farms which sat right atop the moors were subject to a bitter wind the likes of which I've only experienced since in the Alps.

On one occasion I'd been called to see a batch of calves with pneumonia, which is a frustratingly recurrent problem for many farmers in the wintertime. The need to house the animals in a way that keeps them dry, safe, warm and easily accessible for feeding and checking, often means that they are in poorly ventilated buildings, all sharing the same airspace and very effectively recycling and sharing the bacteria and viruses which cause pneumonia. A great many calves can be lost very quickly if action isn't taken when illness breaks out.

This particular farm nestled above the village, along a very narrow track, and its height exposed it to the full force of any inclement weather. The courtyard around which the farm buildings sat and where I had to park was right on the rounded crest of the hill, meaning that I was offered zero protection from a biting wind as I clambered reluctantly out of the cosy comfort of my warm car. At the time the treatment of choice for pneumonia was to give a long-acting and very thick and viscous antibiotic. For the worst affected an injection of an anti-inflammatory would be given to settle the lungs and improve the chances of the calves feeling well enough to eat – and to hopefully keep them alive long enough for the antibiotics to work. I headed into the long barn where the calves were kept and saw that there were about thirty, probably half of which were going to need treatment. Standing to listen and survey for a while before leaping in and stressing the animals, I tried to get an idea of the severity of the outbreak. Animal sheds in winter can be wonderfully serene places that are a delight to the senses. There is the warmth that comes from body heat, the rustle of straw underfoot and the beautiful sound of heavy breath shooting jets of steam from soft, velvety nostrils. Today though, all those gentle nuances were hidden beneath the rattling wheezes and wracking coughs that exploded almost constantly from various animals. The farmer and I moved among the animals slowly so as not to worry and overexert them and I started to gently examine those that were affected as well as checking the apparently normal ones for early signs of illness. When we had a good idea of the number of ill calves I headed out into the numbing wind to get the drugs I needed.

About two minutes later I was standing by the boot of my car trying to draw up the particularly thick injection for the umpteenth calf and I simply couldn't do it. The wind blew straight through me and cut me to my core. I couldn't wear gloves while working with the intricacies of the syringes and needles and my fingers had turned into red and swollen sausages that I couldn't feel anymore. I wondered if I was going to have to pretend that the tears that were threatening to trace their way down my frozen cheeks were because of the wind, not because I was a nine-stone weakling. I finally headed back to the shed and somehow managed to give all the injections with no sign of the tears that had, it seemed, frozen solid before they could fall and give me away. As I drove away I added one more thing to my mental checklist for surviving the learning curve – a portable kit for the essentials so that I didn't have to do the whole thing standing by the car! A simple thing but so stupid to be missing from my armoury.

A few weeks later, in the dead of January, I was starting to feel like a bit of an expert when it came to winter diseases of farm animals. My days were spent racing round the moors from one coughing calf to the next. My muscles were gradually expanding from pitting myself against beef cattle and I even found myself starting to become slightly more impervious to the weather. I was feeling like I had it all under control when Mr Elliot called me into his office and told me I had to go and see a cow with bloat. These are pretty serious cases. A cow can basically be described as a constantly running vat producing a huge quantity of gases that relies solely on an impressive frequency and volume of belching to keep it all under control. If anything blocks the release of this gloriously steady stream of burps the cow will gradually inflate like a Zeppelin and eventually explode. Which is never pretty.

I'd seen several cases of bloat in the months since I started and they are often fairly straightforward to treat, so it was odd that Mr Elliot would take me to one side to tell me about this one. However, it wasn't the cow he wanted to warn me about but the owner. Apparently he was about ninety but Mr Elliot, and indeed most people who knew him, couldn't be sure because he seemed to have been that old forever, so it was really anyone's guess. He was 'a bit frail' and also had 'some sort of heart problem' so I was sombrely warned that I shouldn't expect too much from him because there was a high chance he would simply drop dead. Christ, I thought as I headed out, this was going to be interesting.

The cow in question was one of many that were corralled in a kind of brick-wall affair in the middle of a field. What most vets like when handling animals that weigh half a ton, are not feeling well, and are not particularly keen on being manhandled, is what we call a crush. This is a large, sturdy, metal contraption, which you walk a cow into and which then 'clamps' her into position for want of a better word. Crushes are safe for all concerned and humane for the cow. As I climbed over the gate I cast an eye around at the handling facilities and my heart sank. Inside the brick perimeter was a space about the size of two tennis courts. The cows were huddled under an open shelter where there was concrete to stand on and some protection from the sleet and snow we'd had the last few days. The rest of the 'ground' consisted of a two-foot depth of semi-frozen straw and slurry.

I gingerly climbed down the other side of the gate and put on my best fake smile as I said hello to the tiny slip of a farmer, who wasn't making me feel any less nervous about his prospects of surviving my visit as he wheezed his bronchitic way through what he had planned.

What he proposed was that we somehow separated the cow from the others and moved her over to a wall, where he had loosely tied one end of a metal gate to some old hinges with a couple of bits of bailer twine. We would then coax her towards the hinged end and swing the gate round to pin her in place while I did what I needed to do. What he failed to explain to me was how he, weighing about four stone soaking wet and about as strong as a guinea pig, was going to prevent the enormous and rarely handled beef animal from summarily legging it through him whenever she pleased. But who was I to question the lifelong experience of this wise old man?

The cow in question was pretty easy to distinguish from the rest because she was already swelling quite impressively and her abdomen had already started to dome up at the end of her rib cage as her rumen tried valiantly to take over the rest of her body. It only took about five minutes for my patience and good humour to start to evaporate as we tried between us to separate this one cow from the safety of her herd, hampered by the fact that we had to run after her through knee-high sludge which was like half-frozen quicksand. I'm sure we must have looked like a Benny Hill sketch as we kept on with this farcical chase round the yard. There were cows everywhere. My kingdom for a Border collie, I thought, as I lunged from one direction to the next in another futile round of girl versus cow.

After a lifetime we finally got the ever-expanding beast wedged behind the gate where for a few minutes we all stood defeated, wheezing and puffing from the exertion, cow included. The terrain was probably on our side after all because at least it slowed her down too and I supposed I should count my blessings that the old boy was still breathing. When I finally caught my breath I carefully examined the cow as best I could in the circumstances and decided that the best thing to do would be to get the treatment done and dusted before she too got her breath back and decided to test the strength of the gate and her game old owner. It was only thanks to the fact that her enormous stomach was probably by now compressing her lungs that we managed to contain her at all.

I needed water to mix my anti-bloating potion, which I would then stomach-tube into her to dissipate the lethal bubbly foam that was trapping the gas inside. That was when

I realised that the only water we had was the frozen drinking trough in a dank corner of the enclosure. My already sunken heart dropped a little lower as I realised I was going to have to break the ice and freeze my hands even more. I tried to banish from my memory the fact that cows drinking, or I guessed being pumped full of, near-frozen water can get a fatal freezing and sloughing of their stomach lining. This was not going well.

An age later I'd finally managed to break the ice, get a bucket of water, stir in the powder I needed and was just about to put the stomach tube down the poor creature's gullet when I realised I'd left the pump in the car.

I suppressed a Mr Elliot-esque cacophony of swearing, did an exaggerated sigh and, with barely contained fury at the ill-equipped farmer but mostly at myself for being so stupid, I set off to trudge back through the crap, climb the gate and cross the field to get the pump out of the boot. Because of my black mood I was stomping and huffing and cursing under my breath, which was why I wasn't paying attention to anything else – and which explains why, after about three strides, one powerfully sullen stomp wedged my wellie straight into a foot of cow dung. Before I could engage my brain, I'd taken the next step and then the next with what by now was just a foot with a sock on it, leaving my lonely right wellie waving in the mire, and it was only as my foot plunged up to the knee into the semi-frozen shite that I realised I'd hit rock bottom and that there was nowhere left to go.

By now my blood pressure was threatening to do a Vesuvius as I yanked my lost wellie out and rather redundantly put it back on. A very uncomfortable trudge back to the car did little for my mood and I grabbed the pump and went back again, this time careful to do all my huffy stomping on the frozen grass of the field, not in the bog on the other side of the gate. I pumped the life-saving solution into the beast and wiggled the tube a little to let as much gas escape as I could while it got to work. Job done, we released the cow and I left the farmer with more of the powder to give her later and instructions to call me back if he was at all worried, while secretly praying that I would never have to go back there in my life.

When I left the farm I had undoubtedly saved an animal's life. I might even have done enough to stop an old man dying of overexertion. I tried to tell myself that my little mishap could happen to the most seasoned of vets when faced with such adversity. None of that helped, though, as I limped off, tail between my legs, dignity hanging in tatters and with a soggy, cold and stinking right foot.

Joe and I did at least manage to escape one week of the winter weather by going on a snowboarding holiday. It wasn't as much fun as it sounds for me because after an hour on the slopes I broke my arm and then spent the rest of the week chewing the nails which poked from my plaster cast to stumps, worrying about how to break it to Mr Scary Elliot that I'd be out of action for weeks when I got back. As it turned out he was actually very calm about it when I phoned to pre-warn him and he simply relegated me to solely doing small-animal work for the duration of my incarceration. 'Incarceration' may seem a bit strong but I did begin to feel like I was in prison. I wasn't allowed to drive because of my plaster cast so couldn't get away from the village. I couldn't indulge my passion for surgery for the obvious reason that I needed two hands and I needed to be able to scrub up, and I couldn't take sick leave because I couldn't find a reason that was believable for why I couldn't consult. And so it was that for a good couple of months, until the strength returned to my arm, I found myself imprisoned in our tiny consulting room.

It was during the weeks of my small-animal consulting prison that I became fully aware of another one of Mr Elliot's legendary traits: his driving. Since I'd started at the practice Mr Elliot had had the same pale blue and totally battered Subaru estate. Now farm vets can't be too proud about their cars because the nature of the work makes them smell like a sewer (both the car and, come to think of it, the vets themselves) and leaves all sorts of unmentionables crusted onto the upholstery, but the exterior of this car had prompted a few muttered comments from farmers I'd been to visit. In fact, one had told me that at one time in the car's long and difficult life, and presumably before a major stint of bodywork, there wasn't a single panel on the car that wasn't dented, including the roof.

On my first day back, complete with plaster cast, the car caught my eye as I approached the surgery door. The front had been totally caved in and the bumper and bonnet now resembled a large 'V' with the headlights craned in at an absurd angle. I had a small smile which I tried to wipe off my face as I entered the surgery and I tried to adopt a sombre, funereal air as I asked him solemnly what had happened to his car. The story was preceded by the obligatory huge sigh, several tokes on the ever-present cigarette and sufficient swearing to denote the truly heinous nature of the accident.

It seemed that he had needed to tend to his own sheep because as well as managing a thriving veterinary practice and working inhuman hours, he also ran his own farm. The ground on this occasion had been frozen solid and, instead of going the long way round to his sheep shed, he had opted to go cross-country, as the ground was hard and he had a four-wheel-drive car. He'd happily been driving down the rather steep hill towards this substantial building when he applied the brakes and realised that the ground wasn't just frozen solid but had become a veritable skating rink. The car's brakes locked into a futile death grip on the wheels and he slid the last 30 metres straight into one of the uprights of the huge barn. I tried to make my outburst of laughter into a hearty cough and hurried away to make myself busy.

A few weeks later, when the bulk of the damage had been repaired, I got a close-up-and-personal insight into how the car had come to be such a thing of legend. I was standing in the consulting room listening attentively to a woman telling me about the problems she was having with her dog. The window of the narrow room looked out onto the car park and the consulting table was pushed up against the wall underneath the window sill. As I was telling the client what we should do next a blue movement outside the window caught my eye and I involuntarily turned my head in that direction. Mr Elliot had driven into the car park and was heading straight for the consulting room wall where we were standing. The words dried up in my throat and the client and I stared in motionless disbelief as he sailed towards us without any hint of trying to brake. He coasted merrily up to the building, hit the external wall of the consulting room, ricocheted off a few inches, vigorously pulled the handbrake on and switched off the engine. Having gathered up the papers he needed from the passenger seat, he strolled into the surgery as if absolutely nothing had happened. To this day I don't know if he regularly parked like this in an attempt to save on brake pads or if he had no idea that he'd actually hit the building.

Beside Mr Elliot's misfortunes, in the midst of all the darkness and despair of winter there were four other little things that brightened my days and kept me feeling sane, none of which were planned but fell into my life in what some may call fate and others, being more practically-minded, would call the insatiable need for vets to collect waifs and strays. In fact, gathering forlorn-looking, slightly damaged animals because they feel sorry for them is as much an occupational hazard for vets as having affairs seems to be for Premiership footballers who are married to beautiful, successful women.

I had a wonderful scruffy mongrel called Penny when I was growing up, and when I qualified I had made the conscious decision, even though I've always been a 'dog person', not to get another one yet because of the huge responsibilities that come with owning a dog, not to mention the time and money needed. When my little three-legged cat Charlie had squeezed his way into my life it seemed like the perfect compromise for me. I had the much-loved pet I wanted, and a cat was much more self-sufficient than a dog if I was to be working long hours and travelling to Bideford quite often to see Joe.

In fact it was Joe who started the ball rolling with a phone call one evening. 'Guess what I've got?' he announced excitedly. For a flicker of a second I hoped it wasn't going to be a sexually transmitted disease and quickly gave up trying to guess, which was when he told me that he'd got a puppy. I was astounded because it had always been me who'd hankered after getting a dog while he had never seemed that bothered. He'd been on a farm visit and there they were; a beautiful, leggy farm collie – who had clearly been entertaining a passing stray – and her quite unexpected, unwanted and huge litter of adorable puppies that could best be described as a motley crew. It's anyone's guess what on earth the father was because the pups were long-haired, short-haired, black-and-white, tricolour, blue merle, you name it. The farmer and his wife were lovely people and had welcomed the new batch with an accepting smile, but there was no doubt that they had to be found homes because there is no room on a working farm for a gaggle of half-sheepdogs who may or may not know one end of a sheep from the other.

Joe was bursting with excitement and I felt a pang of jealousy as he described this little bundle of joy he'd adopted and brought home. I couldn't wait to see him and set off the next night after work. He was totally beautiful. Joe had read a boy's adventure book when he was a child which featured a dog called Pan and he had always promised himself that if he ever had a dog that would be what he was called. And so it was that night that I met and instantly fell in love with Pan. I knew immediately that I had to have one too and we convinced ourselves that it would be better for Pan if he had company, so Joe started telling me about the puppies that were left.

I had a paralysing fear that overnight the entire bunch would be snapped up because we couldn't get back to the farm for a couple of days. Eventually the day came and we took Pan with us back to see his mum and his siblings. I'd never had a puppy before because when I was a child my family had always taken on rescue dogs. How was I going to pick? I climbed into the pen and the remaining puppies were ambling about as their mother, seeing the opportunity for a quick break, defied gravity with a deft leap over the partition that contained them. I was squatting down and wondering what criteria I should use to decide when an enormous fat black-and-white bundle waddled over to me, waving an extraordinarily long tail, and clambered onto my knee trying to lick my hands and face. It seemed it wasn't up to me; I'd been chosen and there was nothing I could do but scoop him up and instantly fall in love with him. The name came easily because what black-and-white creatures waddle in such a characteristic way? Badgers. And so it was that Pan and Badger came into our lives and set about destroying our houses, furniture and worldly belongings.

When 'the boys', as they have been known ever since, arrived, Charlie was about six months old. Because of his missing back leg, pronounced limp and diminutive size, I, and everyone who ever saw him, felt sorry for him and I felt very strongly that these boisterous young pups must learn early on to respect the cat and steer clear of him. He was there first and I didn't want him feeling like he'd been ousted in any way, so the boys had a few strongly worded reprimands pretty quickly when bowling around in Charlie's vicinity in those early days.

A couple of weeks after their arrival I was making lunch in the kitchen and the boys were happily playing in the living room. I happened to glance round the doorway, to make sure the poor little kitten wasn't being harassed or flattened, when I saw exactly who was in charge of the situation and was playing me for a fool. Charlie was perched on the back of the settee and the rapidly growing puppies were in a furious pretend fight on the floor beneath him, oblivious to everything except the fun they were having. They rolled apart momentarily and regarded each other, panting to catch their breath before the next round. At this moment Charlie, with lightning speed, ran down the settee, leaned over the edge, swiped Badger clean across the face and returned to where he'd been sitting a split second later as if nothing had happened. I started to go into the room and Charlie knew without a doubt that he'd been caught red-pawed so he just sat there and stared at me as if to say 'prove it'. Trying to reprimand a cat is largely pointless because they are not the subservient please-let-me-please-you types that dogs are and will just regard you with a hostile and rather smug look when told off, so I simply gave Badger a fuss, checked him for bleeding, and retreated to the kitchen in no doubt who was running the house. It seemed the boys and I were going to have to watch out for that one.

I said that there were four additional little things that brightened that winter and the boys were two of them, so you may be wondering what the other two were. One day in February I'd been called out to see a guinea pig which was scratching itself raw and seemed to now be encouraging all its friends to itch too. I arrived at the house and encountered what was probably my first hoarder. There are thousands of animal lovers in our country, probably millions, but there is a small minority who cross the fine line from loving and 'rescuing' animals to hoarding them. Over the years I've seen some horrific cases where this blind love has caused untold suffering in the very animals these people claim to have helped.

At first, the scale of the menagerie wasn't even that obvious. I was shown round the side path to where the multitude of guinea pigs was kept. Having more than one guinea pig is nothing to feel ashamed of and we actively want people to keep these social animals with their own kind, but there were about twenty in various hutches in the garden. I suspected that there was some fairly willy-nilly breeding going on and many of the bunch looked in less than prime condition. It soon became clear that the furious itching, scabs and self-harm was due to a mite infestation that was gripping the colony and spreading gradually amongst them all. Guinea pigs have a really high requirement for vitamin C; it's vital for their immune system and good, healthy skin. Some of the cheaper foods simply don't have enough of the vitamin and it degrades over time so old bags of food or food designed for rabbits just aren't good enough. Over time the lovely little creatures simply lose the ability to fight off the odd parasites they inevitably encounter in bedding and hay and these horrible little mites go haywire, making the guinea pigs tear themselves to shreds like a frantic child with chickenpox.

49

At the time there was virtually nothing available that was licensed for use on guinea pigs so we used to have to use, of all things, a cattle drug. I had a hugely diluted solution with me and all the pigs got a tiny injection to get the mite-killing process started. I drew up a repeat dose for each which could be put on the skin by the owner the following week and told her she needed to address their feeding and get some vitamin supplements in the short term. A third dose would probably be needed to catch any mites that had hatched from eggs left after the initial treatments but I'd be back to check before then anyway. Once the advice had been given and the treatment administered I was invited in for a cup of tea, which it seemed rude to turn down. It was when I entered the house that I realised this kindly lady might be verging on the madder end of the animal-owning spectrum.

There were animals everywhere, with an odd mixture of predators and prey the likes of which I'd never seen. Numerous cats lounged round the place and the accompanying stench hit me like a brick wall as I went into the tiny living room of the small semi-detached house. As my nose became accustomed and my eyes stopped watering I started to notice more and more inhabitants. A few house rabbits were enjoying probably the most stressful existence known to rabbit-kind. There was an enormous vivarium with an equally large python coiled inside it and next to that was a more worryingly empty vivarium, the occupant apparently at large somewhere in the house. I perched on the edge of the sofa starting to wish I hadn't said yes to the tea for fear of all the untold exotic diseases that might come home with me if I ingested anything in the house.

The kindly owner brought me a pallid cuppa and we made chit-chat about her great 'love' of animals, which was when the three-foot monitor lizard that lived in the empty glass case wandered into the room and started looking for its lunch. The woman casually told me that she hadn't really realised it was going to get that big and that it had started to get 'a bit aggressive'. It transpired that it had started to take the odd chunk out of her and had decided that the kittens, which were in never-ending supply in the house, were the perfect size for a midday snack. She confided that she could really do with rehoming the latest batch before the problem of finding them homes was solved by the baby cousin of a Komodo dragon she'd so unwisely bought. I told her I'd see what I could do and made my escape as soon as was reasonably polite.

I phoned one of my favourite clients, Jan, the owner of the goat I had seen on my very first day on the job, who was now a good friend. I seemed to remember she'd mentioned that her brother wanted a cat. She told me he still hadn't found one and that she would go and collect one of the kittens for him. I said I had decided to take one too because I just couldn't bear the thought of their demise in the jaws of the beast. She said she'd collect one for me when she went the next day and bring it over. I requested a tabby male if there was one but said I didn't really mind otherwise.

The next day, as promised, Jan arrived with a little wire carrier containing two minute and gorgeous kittens. A tabby male for the spoilt vet and a bright orange-and-white male for her brother. The thought of taking this tiny creature and launching it, all alone, into my own expanding menagerie seemed so unfair. Jan suggested that I take both kittens and she would get another one for her brother, and so it was that Nigel and Brian joined our merry clan and I had four new bundles of fluff to brighten my winter.

Being more knowledgeable and experienced now, I wouldn't choose to have so many cats because they generally prefer a solitary existence without competition in the shape of other cats, but I've been lucky. My five creatures have always lived in relative harmony. But that's not to say we didn't have our ups and downs.

One of the best things about sharing your life with animals is their varied and wonderful characters. Pan and Badger might have been litter mates but they were very different right from the word go. Pan was the aloof, independent, ever-hungry wolf-lookalike, while Badger was always a mummy's boy. He stuck to my side whenever possible and wedged himself under the back bumper to guard my car if I was on a farm, or under a table or desk when I was at the surgery, wanting to be secure but banging his nobbly head about a hundred times a day whenever he got out from whatever he was hiding under.

From quite early on it was obvious that neither dog had inherited any herding instinct or skills whatsoever from their mother, but Pan did show very early what we would medically term 'bonkers Border collie' traits. Dulverton being the very small place it was, there were limits to what was on offer for entertainment, but just up the road from the icebox I was living in there was a great pub, which held a lot of appeal on many a dark winter evening. The pub was archetypal rural British and had just the right balance of cosiness and dim lighting combined with the inexplicable but seemingly obligatory array of stuffed animals adorning the walls.

The dogs have always been superbly behaved, mostly through their superior part-collie brains rather than anything to do with the wonders of my teaching abilities, and were always good when in places like the local pub. They would both sit obediently under the table and generally be what we would call 'dog ambassadors'. However, Joe and I soon realised that this was only in pubs that didn't have a dartboard. The evening started off fairly normally, but then we decided to head into the public bar because it was too crowded to sit down in the 'posh' bar. We'd settled ourselves at the table when a couple of the locals got up to play darts. The first couple of thuds went relatively unnoticed and then Pan's ears pricked up and he was straight up on his haunches, head up and as alert as we'd ever seen him. He waited patiently while the man collected his darts and then watched as the next one stepped up to the oche. The arm came back and as the dart let fly Pan leapt to his feet in excitement. He had a fire in his eye you wouldn't believe, his mouth opened in glee and his huge tongue lolled out as the next arrow found its target. The boys were never on leads and as he jumped up to join in we called him back with bemused smiles on our faces. 'SIT!' we said firmly and he parked his bum without taking his eyes off the player, but two seconds later he was on all fours again running on the spot and squealing with each dart's flight.

We apologised profusely to the distracted pair but they smiled good-naturedly just like us because no one had ever seen anything like it. We even tried the lure of a forbidden crisp,

Pan's main love in life (until he discovered darts) being food, but he gave the proffered titbit a split-second glance over his shoulder and totally ignored it. Unbelievable. He was utterly transfixed and couldn't contain himself, tearing backward and forward between the oche and the board, panting furiously with the maddest look on his face you could imagine. By now we were crying with laughter, which didn't really help our attempts to control our loony dog, but the game continued without too much hindrance. In fact the players were more concerned about the odd dart that hit the wires of the board and bounced out at random and dangerous angles around this crazed beast. When a dart landed on the floor it became clear that the excitement was not a game of fetch. He had no interest whatsoever in the objects when they were still, it was just the flight he wanted to watch.

To this day Pan has amused hundreds of people in pubs all across the country with his fascination with the dartboard. If ever you wanted to see a dog adopting the pose of 'His Master's Voice' with dedicated loyalty, it is Pan when no one is playing darts. He can be found sitting directly below the board, unmoveable, and ever hopeful whenever someone walks past that they will have a game just for him. On occasions too numerous to count, especially where we live now, the locals actually go to play darts just for Pan. It seems that no one can ignore those doleful eyes that follow you as you walk past with a pleading look that says, 'Please, sir, just the one game of 301.' But of course, as any addict will tell you, one game is never enough and so poor Pan is always left wanting. On one brilliant outing we went to a pub that had a circular, pictured mirror. Pan assumed it was a dartboard and took up his position, staring alternately at the mirror above his head and likely-looking passers-by, no doubt wondering why no one would oblige.

In the early days when Joe and I were living separately, so did the boys for the most part. They were together nearly every night as we commuted one way or the other, but during the working day Pan would be with his 'dad' and Badger with me. It wasn't long before Joe asked me if I could have Pan for a couple of days because he had to go away and couldn't take Pan with him. I was more than happy to oblige because the boys loved being together and they kept each other occupied. They were about six months old now and all my farmers were used to Badger ambling about the place while I did my work so I could see no problem with there being two of them. What I didn't realise was that my softie boyfriend had not instilled in Pan quite the farm etiquette that I had assumed.

On a glorious morning in March I'd gone to see a lovely farm client of ours who was having the age-old winter problem of calf pneumonia. With many of his animals affected I knew it would be a long visit. I checked with him about the boys and with his blessing released them to explore while I grabbed what I needed from the boot and went into the dark confines of the large shed to see the calves.

As I emerged into the bright, crisp sunlight about an hour later the farmer was just on his way in to see me. He looked a bit uncomfortable, and before I could say anything, he uttered the immortal line, 'Your new dog's just mauled my wife's two remaining hens.' I felt the colour drain from my face. I looked round and saw my angelic Badger in his usual position under the back bumper of the car, and then Pan appeared looking very happy with himself indeed and clearly with no idea that he had done anything at all wrong. I spluttered a profuse apology and asked what had happened. The farmer had found one bird dead and the other maimed badly enough that he had had to wring its neck. I was absolutely speechless. How could a vet have such an animal? I'm sure he could tell I was mortified and said with a cheeky smile on his face that he was bloody sick of the chickens and had wanted his wife to get rid of them for ages so Pan had done him a favour. He was letting me off the hook, I knew. I offered compensation, which he declined, but it did nothing for the numb feeling I had in the pit of my stomach.

That night when I spoke to Joe on the phone I was livid that he could have allowed me to let such a murderous beast loose on a farm without telling me what he was like. Of course it wasn't really Joe's fault because he did much more small-animal work than me, and so Pan simply hadn't had the farm time that Badger had had. Also, Pan was so much more outgoing, and even if Badger had any lethal tendencies he was just too scared to get out from under the car to act on them!

A couple of days later when the fowl-killing beast of Bideford was safely back at his dad's house, I was at the surgery writing up some notes when a brother and sister team from one of our farms popped in to settle up their account. I smiled cheerily at them and was met with a black look and a scowl that quickly wiped the smile from my face. 'While you were at the farm the other day your dog killed our dad's prize drake.' Oh crikey. I'd been out to see them just before the hen-hunting incident and had no idea. That was clearly where Pan had discovered he had quite a taste for blood. There was nothing I could say except that I was sorry and that it would never happen again. This time there was clearly going to be no easy smile and awkward laughter to gloss over the heinous crime. Their steely looks left no doubt about how totally outraged the family was, their dad in particular, and rightly so. I have always been the sort of person who will torture myself endlessly about the smallest perceived slight against anyone, even when it's only imagined. Add to that my despair when I see badly behaved dogs or irresponsible owners and my horror at any hint of animal suffering and you can imagine the inner turmoil that kept me awake that night. It was decided; I told Joe that Pan couldn't come on any more visits with me, full stop. Hopefully his livestock-slaughtering days had come and *very* quickly gone.

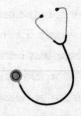

Chapter 3

This is a man's world, but it wouldn't be nothin'...

1991, the year that I went to Bristol vet school, was the first year that the ratio of girls to boys became fifty–fifty. The veterinary profession was, until then, a very male-dominated one but that had gradually started to change and my year marked the tipping point. By 2010 it was more like eighty per cent women who were going to vet school with a smattering of lucky boys. Surrounded by intelligent beauties, they must have thought that all their birthdays had come at once!

At the same time, it's true that farm work has been in serious decline for a number of years as small farms have gone out of business. With the changing face of agriculture and the huge increase in people's love of pets, the shift in the balance of work has turned hugely towards the small-animal market. But when I qualified in 1996 there was then, as there is now, no reason at all for women not to be just as capable and successful in farm and equine work as men. The fact is that with modern technology the days of hauling calves out of cows with brute force or, God forbid, a tractor, have long gone and hopefully cows are much better off for it. On Exmoor, where sheep-work was in abundance, there are many benefits to being a woman, the greatest advantage being our small hands. When you're trying to manipulate a small lamb in a small birth canal, having muscles like Popeye and hands like spades does little to help your corner. When I got to Exmoor the vast majority of farmers were more than used to seeing female vets and I virtually never encountered intolerance because of my gender. Apart, that is, from one classic case.

The call came at about four in the morning as we were starting to climb out of the depths of winter and into the very welcome onset of spring. Let's be honest; there isn't a person on earth who actually relishes being woken up at some ungodly hour from a deep slumber, but these occasions do let you see the best the world has to offer. I've never been a morning person and, no matter how often I see a beautiful sunrise and think that I really should get up sometimes just to see them, I never quite manage to actually haul my sorry self out of bed.

It was still dark when I left to go and see a cow which was having difficulty calving, and it was a farm I'd not been to yet in the six months or so I'd been working on Exmoor. When I got called to my first ever calving I was absolutely petrified because I thought, 'If this farmer has been calving cows for thirty years and he can't figure out what's wrong then what the hell good am I going to do?' The fact is, though, that many farmers, maybe from bitter experience or just good sense, know that if everything doesn't feel just so then it's best to call the vet or it can end in disaster, not only for your animals but your wallet too. And so I soon learned that I did in fact have something to offer these largely lovely folk.

Being involved in any animal's birth is one of the most enduringly wonderful things that I have ever come across in all my years in practice. It may sound clichéd but no matter how often you've done it or been there, there is nothing on the planet that compares to seeing a newborn anything nuzzling in to its mother. Equally, nothing quite matches the tragedy of those births that go wrong.

And so it was, as ever, with some trepidation that I drove to the farm, not knowing the set-up they had, the knowledge or expertise of the farmer or what I would ultimately find when I first felt inside the cow. The first hint of dawn was just lightening the sky as I arrived and I drove down the little track to the barn where a wiry and fairly grim-faced man was standing. There is a brilliant German phrase which is *ein Gesicht wie sieben Tage Regenwetter haben*, which means 'to have a face like seven days of rain', and this pretty much summed him up. There was a gruff hello followed by a no-niceties escort to the stall where the cow was labouring away. On the way the farmer explained how he had been trying to calve her for some time and he usually had no problems at all and he didn't really want to call us and generally made me feel about as welcome as an unexpected rash on your nether regions.

It wasn't until I started getting my calving top on and sorting out my kit that he unleashed his main reason for not wanting me there. Casually leaning on the wooden partition to the cow's stall, he offered no help or tea or anything at all for that matter except an unceasing diatribe about how, no offence intended of course, he just didn't think that women were up to the job. This wasn't a simple one-off comment; he kept on and on. After about five minutes he turned sideways to lean his back against the wooden partition of the stall and consequently had his back turned to me and his cow. With arms folded and one wellie crossed comfortably over the other he carried on happily ranting about how he had no problem with women in general and he didn't begrudge them equal pay or good jobs or any of those things (which probably meant secretly he was gobsmacked we'd been given the vote) but that for physical work like this there was no substitute for the good old-fashioned strength and size that men had to offer. We women were just too damn weedy to be of any use to a farmer like him. If he couldn't calve the cow then there was no way a woman could and he was pretty sure that eventually I'd have to phone one of my male partners to bail me out so I could get back to painting my nails or whatever it was he thought I should be doing with my time.

I'd been on the farm for literally about fifteen minutes when I interrupted the deluge of verbal diarrhoea to say that I was done and I'd be going on my way. He turned to look at me like a rabbit in the headlights and then, unspeaking and open-mouthed, looked down at the floor by my feet where two perfect twin calves lay, shaking their sticky heads to free their glorious big ears as the cow was turning towards them with the mothering instinct that millennia of evolution had given her.

He opened and closed his mouth a couple of times and still nothing was forthcoming. I used the rare silence to tell him that he had in fact been pulling one leg of each calf thinking that it was one animal and chose to leave out my preferred end to the sentence, which was 'you idiot, sexist, halfwit'. All I'd done was simply feel that there were two, push one of the eager young things back so that one could come fully into the birth canal and then pull them out one at a time. The truly great part was that, being twins, they were so small that I hadn't even had to use any leverage in the shape of the usual calving jack and had simply pulled them both out – with my puny girl arms!

I gathered my belongings, said a cheery goodbye as I climbed into the car and drove away with the sight of him in the rear-view mirror, still standing there staring after me with his mouth open, forever etched into my memory. When I reached a safe distance I let go of the huge beaming smile that I'd been bursting with the entire time and started laughing so hard I had to pull over. I sat in the car grinning like an idiot on a beautiful hillside and watched the sun come up over the moors. I suddenly knew in that instant that all my hard work had paid off. I'd really made it. It was a rare and perfect moment and one that I will always cherish.

That's not to say that some of the unique needs of being a woman haven't left me a little red-faced in the job. On another equally unforgettable occasion I'd been scheduled to do a routine visit to another one of our ancient clients. I don't know if it's something in the water or just being hardened up by good, lifelong physical labour, but we had quite a few farmers on our books who were well into their seventies and eighties and still going strong, working on the farm every day. This particular farmer was one of those men of myth that everyone uses when they are trying to excuse bad habits in themselves like smoking, drinking and a bad diet by saying they know of someone who hasn't fallen foul of such vices. This man had smoked a multitude of cigarettes seemingly every day since birth, ate a fried breakfast every day of his life and no doubt saw off every evening with a shot or two of strong whisky before bed and was showing no signs of giving up the ghost anytime soon.

I'd been to the farm a couple of times before for minor things but this would be a longer visit for the purpose of disbudding and castrating a batch of young calves. Many people don't realise that most cattle are born with the potential to grow horns and later in life, with a lot of muscle behind them, those horns can be at best a nuisance and at worst downright dangerous. To stop the problems that are inherent with horns we 'disbud' calves at a young age. The process is pretty straightforward: it involves an injection of local anaesthetic near the base of the soft little horn bud and then, once the area is numb, a hot iron implement is used to burn away the bud tissue so that it never develops into a horn. Apart from the rather acrid smell of burning hair the procedure is painless and causes very little upset to the animal. It sounds brutal, but it isn't, and I can assure you that trying to remove fully formed horns from adult bulls is no picnic for either the poor blighter trying to saw through four inches of pretty solid horn or the animal who by now has become rather attached to them!

I was looking forward to the visit because it was one of those lovely farms where the farmer's wife would always have laid on a little something at the house for me no matter how quick the visit might be. On this occasion I'd taken all my kit and the heavy gas cylinder with the disbudding iron on top over to the old tumbledown stalls where the calves had been brought in and were waiting. The lovely old farmer was there, as was his son or grandson (I never did get to grips with the family tree), both looking expectantly at me as I got the tools of my trade together. The iron needed time to heat up to its efficient best so I reached confidently into my trouser pocket to get my lighter out and hoiked it out of an awkward corner with some gusto. The lighter freed itself with some force and brought with it a great and colourful rainbow cascade of tampons which rained down into the tangled straw at my feet. There were a few distinct moments where these wonderfully antiquated gents didn't know where to look as I dived into the straw, scrabbling around for my not-so-secret-anymore bounty and started stuffing them back into any pocket I could reach, desperately trying to pretend that they might be anything besides items of the so awfully named 'feminine hygiene' variety. Bless them, I'm sure being farmers they were perfectly au fait with everything to do with reproduction in all species including ours, but they could see I was mortified so after a couple of embarrassing throat-clearings they suddenly found very urgent things to be busying themselves with while I regained my composure. These days, my timid nature long behind me, I'm sure we would have had a great laugh about it but I knew my face was scarlet as I lit the flame on the disbudding iron and on that day, at least, I wasn't celebrating my gender in quite the same way as before.

On the whole, our farm clients were at ease with female vets and I really felt very welcome wherever I went. But sometimes it's not just your gender that can leave people a little disgruntled when you appear for the first time and want to try to help one of their beloved animals. Looks can also present an obstacle. The vast majority of our large-animal work was cattle and sheep but we did tend to the needs of a few horses too. Some belonged to farmers and their families, we had a couple of small riding stables on the books and we had a few clients with large and pretty flash liveries where beautiful, noble-looking and no doubt expensive creatures resided. It was to one of the latter places that I was called early that spring to see a horse with colic. The very mention of the word colic strikes fear into many a horse owner but it is a very general term simply meaning abdominal pain. The causes are extremely varied, from a simple spasm of the guts, which is easily treated, to life-threatening bowel obstructions which can kill horses in a matter of hours without swift and decisive surgical intervention. Hence the fear and panic when a horse starts kicking its belly and sweating and generally shouting in horse, 'Help me! I'm too young for the glue factory!'

As I drove down the long and impressive drive that led onto the property, I could see the extensive, perfectly manicured fields and stables spread out behind the mansion, for want of a better word, that dominated the foreground. The financial worth of an animal must never enter into any clinical decisions or dictate importance in any way, but when I know I'm about to treat an animal that's potentially worth thousands of pounds it undoubtedly heaps a little more pressure on my narrow shoulders. Having only been qualified about eight months, I gulped as I parked the car and headed for the front door. I rang the bell and waited patiently, having a sneaky look round at the impressive set-up. After a few seconds a very tall, angular and rather overbearing man answered the door, leaned slightly towards me and literally looked down on me from a great height with a quizzical look on his face. I gave him my brightest smile and said I'd come to see his horse. He simply stared at me, totally unspeaking, for so long that I felt I should repeat myself so I said again, 'I've come to see your horse?' with a slight questioning air because I was suddenly wondering if I was barking up the wrong tree or if I'd come to the wrong place entirely.

Again there was an unnerving silence while he just stared at me. I was starting to feel distinctly uncomfortable. Was I speaking a foreign language? Was this an asylum where the mentally unbalanced were allowed to answer the door? There didn't seem to be much else to do but say, more emphatically this time, 'Did you ring the vet's about a horse with colic?' and finally he straightened up and said, 'Yeeees?' as if he now wasn't sure whether he had or not.

'I'm the vet,' I tried again.

'No you're not.'

This was unexpected. 'Yes, I *am*.'

'You're too young to be a vet.'

'I *am* a vet!' I wasn't sure what else I could do. When you leave vet school you don't get issued with a laminated badge proving you're qualified. I felt like I needed a leather wallet with a police-style gold shield that I could whip out with a flourish and flash in his face but as it was I had nothing except my word. This had never happened to me before. I didn't really know whether I looked young or not. I mean, I was only twenty-four so I *was* pretty young. What else did he expect me to do?

After my final firm assertion he just kind of caved in, grabbed his coat from the hook by the door and said 'right' in much the same way as John Cleese would have done at his harassed best in *Fawlty Towers*, and strode off towards the stables. I half skipped and half ran to keep up with him, trying for the life of me not to look like a schoolchild skipping in the playground and all the while desperate to pull an immature face towards his retreating back. The pressure was definitely on and I prayed to the gods of good fortune to let me save the day by astounding him with my clinical acumen and mature handling of his beast. And, for the love of Pete, to let me hit the vein the first time if the poor creature needed intravenous drugs.

Luckily for me the rest of the visit was a dream. The colic was a simple one, the horse was impeccably behaved instead of being half a ton of needle-shy lunacy and my hand was steady as a rock as I expertly slid my needle into the huge jugular that so kindly presented itself to me with a neon sign overhead saying 'this way to the vein'.

When I left I hoped the man had at least started to believe I'd actually graduated from vet school and I pictured him heading back home to his wife all the time shaking his head with an air of disbelief. He wanders into the kitchen, lets out a big sigh and she turns to look at him expectantly as he rubs his chin and starts muttering about how not only policemen but now the bloody vets all look too young.

I think a number of factors contributed to what happened next as I drove back to the surgery, one of them being that I was caught up in this reverie, others being that the road was wet from the recent rain, the sun had come out and was glaring off the slick tarmac, I was starving and rushing to get back to the surgery to inhale a sandwich, but mostly I suspect that some road planning idiot had failed to put one of those rather helpful whacking great black-and-white arrows that warn you about impending doom on the deceptive bend that I was approaching at about fifty miles an hour.

I say deceptive because it lulled me into a false sense of security as it started as a very negotiable bend and then chuckled to itself and hardened off into a grand prix turn. I slammed the brakes on, aquaplaned and very possibly accelerated straight across the other lane, sailed up the steep verge and was brought to a very sudden and effective stop by a six-foot hedge. The road I had until very recently been travelling on was the main route across the moors towards Minehead and had logging lorries going up and down it all day. It struck me as I sat in the hedge, feeling rather dazed, to say the least, that I was more than a bit lucky that I hadn't ended up wedged under the bumper of a juggernaut. Feeling remarkably calm and collected, I went to get out and found that I was very snugly ensconced in the hedge indeed. I battered the driver's door against the robust plant enough to squeeze out and wandered onto the roadside to survey the damage. Yes, the car was definitely in a hedge and quite positively so. There didn't seem to be much I could do except hope to flag down a passing car, at which very moment, would you believe, a taxi came round the corner. Probably not his usual manner of gaining custom, he very kindly raised an eyebrow and pulled straight over. I was awash with all sorts of natural fight-or-flight biological chemicals like adrenaline and I don't think I fully comprehended what had happened but the look on his face made it quite clear how the accident looked from the outside world. Basically there was a crumpled car a good few feet above ground level teetering in a hedge and a young woman wandering about in the road looking like she was away with the fairies. He jumped out and put a steadying arm towards me. 'Are you ok?' he asked.

'Fine,' I dreamily replied, 'could you give me a lift back to Dulverton please?'

I can't remember what we talked about, or even if we talked at all, on the ten-minute drive back to town. Yet again I found myself awash with hysterical, post-traumatic tears once safely back in the surgery and in the warm and wonderful embrace of Mary and Bretia. As you may have gathered by now, there were in fact quite a few instances in my first few months in practice which had me in tears. I've never been under any illusions that I'm like a rock when it comes to my emotions. My mum has often told me that even the theme music to *Lassie* made me cry when I was a child, but I had expected shed tears to result from lost animals, not from being kicked, frozen and crashed! I resolved to stop being such a wuss and 'man up'. Once I'd composed myself I set off to the local garage to see about getting my car retrieved. I was starting to think I shouldn't have been quite so smug about Mr Elliot's driving and the state of his car.

Andy, the man at the garage, said they'd go and get the car and have it back with me as soon as possible. Clearly neither of us had quite appreciated how thoroughly I'd 'parked' the car because about an hour later he came back to report that they'd had to call a garage in Minehead because the car was so impaled that it needed lifting up and off the hedge to get the branches out of the engine compartment. In the meantime they gave me a courtesy car and I tried to get on with business.

It took about three weeks to get my car back. Andy explained that the reason I'd not suffered even a single niggle from the force of the impact was that my lovely car had been designed to totally cave in to absorb it for me. Consequently, twelve hundred pounds later, the chassis had been straightened, the bonnet and front end replaced and, I imagine, quite a lot of foliage removed from various bits of the engine. The car looked brand new and *clean*! I've always viewed car cleaning as an absolute waste of time and energy so seeing my car clean was like having it brand new all over again, especially seeing as after only a few hours of farm work it was always full of used rectal gloves, body fluids and faeces and smelt like a septic tank. I promised myself I would try to keep it nice this time and proudly set off for my visits.

About a week later I was high on the moors at a farm which was down a very narrow track and had been called to see a cow which was having problems 'getting into calf'. This means she wasn't getting pregnant as expected, not that she was futilely trying to climb into a young bovine. The reason that vets always seem to have their arms inside cows (apart from the warmth) is that it is the best way to feel all the structures in the abdomen. You can diagnose dozens of problems by feeling around, from the voluminous stomachs right down to the ovaries and uterus and even, once practised in the art, tell if the ovaries are producing eggs or just sitting there with their feet up having a cup of tea because they've lost track of time.

After a thorough internal examination I had ascertained that the cow in question had very little happening on the ovary front, so she needed to have a hormone injection to start her ovulatory processes going. This would then hopefully make her cast an eye over the resident bull and think, 'Hmm..., maybe I would.' I'd parked the car in the large courtyard which was miraculously spotless on this rare pristine farm and had got out the things I needed, leaving the boot resting down but not latched shut.

Having given the cow her injection and told the farmer when we ought to see her again, we were enjoying some polite chit chat when a man came round the corner looking a little worried and asked whose Peugeot was parked round the corner. Oh no. Having identified me as the owner he very apologetically explained that he had just BACKED A LIBRARY into it. What! We trooped round the corner and, sure enough, there was my little car, back end caved in, boot hydraulics sheared off and a bloody great yellow Mercedes *library* idling nearby, looking menacing and very pleased with itself.

Back to Andy I went, and I was starting to see how a small village could sustain such a prosperous garage. Between me and Mr Elliot they probably didn't need anyone else. I was very conscious that I was starting to look like an inept woman driver so I had to be very firm in my assertion that I wasn't even in the car when the library hit it. I wondered if my insurance company were going to buy this one. If only the cameras had been there, I'd have had proof.

Vets in Practice turned out, to my surprise, to be enormously popular and I think that many of the viewers assumed that the cameras were there all the time (much like the dreadful *Big Brother* house in more recent years), but this wasn't the case. The crew would come for a week or a few days at a time and just hope that interesting stuff happened while they were there. It was always great if we got a good case but, as with any job, there are inevitably days and days where only the most dull and routine things happen. And with Sod's Law so often intervening, the most incredible cases would often pop up on the exact day the cameras had gone home. When they were with us, though, it was the job of the researcher to plough through the op sheets, appointment lists and visit book and try to pick which cases (and clients) would turn out to be TV gems and which ones would be a waste of the licence fee. This was of course a learning curve.

When they first started with us virtually everything got filmed, whether it was a slightly fishy-smelling Corgi having its anal glands squeezed (you really don't want to know) or a heroic, lifesaving Caesarean section. The crew would ask me roughly what I thought some of the cases might entail and I'd try to help by guessing as best I could but, to be honest, I didn't really have much experience at that stage either. After the crew had been coming to us for a few months, we'd been standing in the little office where the visit book resided when I overheard Emma, the researcher, talking to Amanda, the director. They were poring over the book and trying to decide what they would shadow me for and what they would drink tea through.

'What about this calf with pneumonia?' said Amanda, no doubt hoping there might be a life-threatening angle they could make out of it.

'No,' said Emma, with total confidence, 'that'll just need some Micotil and Zenecarp.' And she was right. Then they just carried on looking at the book as if this was the most natural thing in the world for her to say. I stood mute in the corner wondering how she knew that and fleetingly wondered if she would go on the visit for me if I told her the doses and gave her some wellies.

This became harder for me to ignore later that day when it came to afternoon surgery. Just beforehand, the same editorial procedure had happened with the appointment list.

'What about this dog with vomiting and diarrhoea?' said Amanda.

'Well, it will probably just need starving overnight then feeding a bland diet like boiled chicken and rice and maybe, if it's got a temperature, some Synulox,' said my new nemesis, Emma. (I should point out that we don't often advise withholding food these days, but back then it was indeed the done thing.) I was about to interrupt to pedantically point out that there were *actually* a number of serious diseases and conditions which could present themselves as a simple case of vomiting and diarrhoea, *actually*, when the bloody know-it-all added, 'But sometimes there is more going on so we should probably film that one.' Bitch. I was starting to have an inkling that my five years at vet school might not have actually been necessary. It seemed that Emma, having observed veterinary practice for all of about twenty days in total, could probably have blagged her way through ninety per cent of my work completely undetected.

The problem for me at the time was that I desperately wanted there to be something I could add. How could she know everything I was going to say and do before I did it? Later that afternoon the tiny consulting room was packed with the owner, the dog, me, the cameraman and the sound man. There simply wasn't room for Amanda or Emma but as I finished examining the dog I knew they would both see the footage and know the outcome, so I didn't want to say it but I had no choice. As the words started to come out, I detected the faintest hint of a snigger from one of the crew.

'I'm pleased to say that there doesn't seem to be anything seriously wrong with him and I suspect he's just scavenged something out of a bin or on a walk and has an upset stomach. What I'd like you to do is starve him overnight and then tomorrow feed him a bland diet of boiled chicken and rice.' It took all my maturity not to lean out of the room and say to Emma, 'It didn't need Synulox, actually, and, for your information, there are other antibiotics we sometimes use!'

I can't really say too much against the poor lass because after a few weeks of being filmed I had also started to pick up bits of filming lingo and found myself reminding the crew about continuity or some other such filming must. On the rare instances I could remind Emma about some such trivial point I could have a little private moment of revenge to myself. I must, however, admit that, despite her uncanny vetting abilities and my rather competitive nature, we did become firm friends and have remained so to this day.

Being filmed was in many ways a very odd experience for an ordinary member of the public like me. I was absolutely astounded when I was first recognised in a street away from where I lived. Being someone who doesn't watch much television, I simply found it impossible to believe that, after I'd been shown for just a few slots in one series, people would be able to pick me out of a crowd with total certainty as 'that vet off the telly'. It seems strange in hindsight that that has now become the norm for me even years after the programme finished. Of course it would be nice if someone remembered my actual name rather than just wanting to know about Trude, the stunning Scandinavian megastar of the show. I suppose I should be glad she didn't work at the same practice as me or I might never have had any clients!

When I lived in Dulverton and the television programme was aired, Joe and I started having press articles written about us, which was both enormously exciting and enormously weird, and it brought some pressure when we had to live up to headlines like 'Is this Britain's most perfect couple?' (As we'll see later, 'no' turned out to be the answer to that one.) We were really only very minor celebrities but then one glorious Saturday we read an article which made us realise we'd made it to the big time. Up until that point we'd appeared in local papers and had a couple of column inches in the tabloids, but that day we happened to see the review of the previous night's television in *The Guardian* (yes, a broadsheet!) and noticed not only that *Vets In Practice* was discussed but that Joe himself had been singled out for a mention. The programme the night before had featured Joe having to see a young child, his mother and a rather moribund hamster. Many vets live in more fear of these tiny rodents than they do of any forty-kilo, highly trained prison guard dog. You can muzzle, drug and sit on the latter, but hamsters will bite you every time if they feel the need. Holding them tightly by the scruff of the neck sometimes works but some of the most practised vet-savaging little blighters can turn bodily round in their own skin and get you anyway. Add to this the fact that they are virtually always the pets of small, sweet, heart-meltingly cute children who look at you with their huge, pleading, Bambi eyes to save their beloved, butter-wouldn't-melt-in-his-mouth Fluffy. Then pile onto that the fact that tiny creatures like hamsters and budgies, who are eaten by other animals in the wild, have a habit of promptly dying as soon as anything as scary as a vet even thinks about trying to examine them.

On this occasion Joe certainly hadn't needed to worry about the hamster biting him because the creature looked like he was lining the bucket up to kick it and was tucked up trying to leave his mortal coil in peace when he had been brought into a surgery, had a camera pointed at him and had a young and eager vet try to save his life by giving him an injection. As the tiny drop of liquid left the syringe the hamster popped his clogs very decisively, and instantly hung there, limp on the end of the needle. There was a second of awful silence where the horror of the situation sunk in before Joe, not having many other options, muttered that the hamster was dead and put him back in his box, smiled awkwardly at the small child and practically shouted 'Next!' as the poor duo were hustled from the room. It was heartbreaking television and probably didn't show Joe's usually caring and warm bedside manner at its best, which is probably what had prompted the television reviewer to write the immortal words, '...and then Joe, the hamster-murdering bastard...'. Oh yes, we knew we were famous then. Obviously, I hadn't been mentioned at all but I was happy to bask in the reflected glory of being the *Guardian*-mentioned, hamster-murdering bastard's girlfriend. It was tenuous, I know, but for all I knew this was our one series and our fifteen minutes of fame. As it turned out, no one could have guessed just how popular it was going to be.

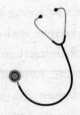

Chapter 4

To sleep, perchance to dream

As spring fully ousted winter from the moors, everything started to come back to life and what were beginning to feel like permanent browns and greys started to yield to a glorious array of greens. Just as I've never been a morning person, I am equally not a winter person. I don't mind winters if they are crisp, frosty, beautiful, sunny and, most importantly, short. England, however, rarely delivers this kind and by February I always find myself wondering if it will ever end. Will I ever see blue sky again? I heard someone on the radio once comment that living in England is like living in a Tupperware box because the sky looks like a Tupperware lid for so much of the time. It's a brilliant analogy but I wish I'd never heard it because now it's all I can think about on those unending grey days when the sun seems to have lost the energy to even lift itself into the sky let alone penetrate the murk hanging over us.

With every spring I feel like I'm reborn. I seem to be able to breathe more deeply, the light mornings give me as much oomph as I'll ever muster to get out of bed and my mood lightens in synchrony with the days. Of all the places I've lived I think this was most noticeable in Exmoor, probably because I was outside working through the winter so bore the full brunt of the weather day after day. I spent long hours driving across the moors to get to our furthest farms and those moors are such a bleak place to be on any but the brightest of days. I soon realised why so many literary and film greats are centred around wild, isolated moorland locations. I used to dread getting stranded and, having had a ridiculously overactive imagination from birth, I used to scare myself witless on dark nights when I was on call.

Being on call is one of the oddest double-edged swords of our job. On one hand you are often doing interesting, adrenalin-fuelled work, which is what you signed up for in the first place, but on the flip side it can make you feel manacled, resentful and stuck in an odd limbo-like frame of mind where you are neither at work nor able to relax. The job in Dulverton didn't pull any punches when it came to the rota and with the onset of spring things got a whole lot worse.

Rotas vary hugely between practices and I believe the profession is in a period of flux at the moment. We are moving from the days of very mixed and often basic work, with little or no comeback if things go wrong, into a period of advanced technology and high expectations. With veterinary knowledge expanding at a rate of knots and surgical and medical advances in step with human medicine, it is becoming harder and harder to be a jack of all trades and still do the job justice. A culture of litigation has upped the stress, the substance abuse and, tragically, the suicide rate among vets. With increasing pressures and workloads, and also changing attitudes to what constitutes a sensible work-life balance (or work-liver balance as my great friend John calls it), more and more practices are outsourcing their on-call rota to specialist emergency centres, or at least making allowances for time off after being on call. But of course all this depends on where you are and in 1997 on Exmoor there were just the three of us, miles from anywhere, with no one to back us up except each other.

Mr Elliot, trooper that he was, did two nights every week in return for not having to do any Friday nights, which left Martin and me to do one night each every week and alternate Fridays. Then we had to have two of us on every Saturday morning to cover farm and small-animal work and then one vet to be on call for the rest of the weekend until Monday morning. What this boiled down to was that I only got one complete weekend off every six weeks. Added to this was the astounding fact that there was no extra fee for calling us out (as is common practice just about everywhere this side of Mars), which meant that it was very tempting for a minority of our clients to call us out at their own convenience if they couldn't make it in for the surgery times. I remember one Sunday afternoon around three o'clock I was phoned by a very worried couple because their dog was choking and they thought it might have something stuck in its throat. In the background I could hear this terrible retching and gagging and agreed immediately to meet them at the surgery as soon as they could get there. When they arrived and I started to examine the dog, I was going through the history as I did so and asked them when exactly it had started. That was when I got the astounding answer that it had started some thirty-odd hours previously on Saturday morning, but they had had a wedding to go to so had waited until they returned to get the poor creature examined. Times like this as a vet can be, shall we say, more than a little frustrating! As it transpired the dog had quite a bad case of kennel cough and didn't have anything actually lodged in its windpipe but it could have been very much worse.

I have to admit I was struggling a bit with the rota and over the months since starting I'd started to get more than a little paranoid and superstitious about normal, everyday aspects of life. For example, it seemed that every time I got in the bath I'd get called out. Every time my dinner was half-cooked I'd get called out and it would be too far gone not to be ruined. No matter how late I stayed up or waited for it to 'quieten down', I would get called out just as I got my clothes off, dived under the ever-cold covers and turned off the light. By spring, when it was my turn on call I'd stopped eating anything except bread, I'd stopped washing and I had started sleeping fully clothed! You can imagine that by the end of a weekend on call I was pretty hungry and tired, not to mention the fact that I didn't exactly smell of roses, either. And *then* lambing started.

I realise I'm about to sound very old indeed to many of you, but when I qualified mobile phones were only just starting to appear. It's mind-boggling how much has changed since then. I didn't even have a mobile until after I left university. The first model I got had a talktime of eight whole minutes and a standby battery life of six hours. Oh yes, it was state of the art! Where I lived it was totally useless, and not just because of its rather unimpressive features. Mobile coverage was patchy at best in major cities 'in those days', so we didn't have a hope up and down all over the moors. In fact we couldn't even have the beepers which many of my friends had for their jobs for the same reason: the impenetrable countryside shunned any form of communication that wasn't physically attached to something by a wire. This meant that we used to rely solely on a trusty old answering machine, and remember that back then this had a tape in it, not a digital, hard-drive style memory. When I got called to any of our furthest farms I would make sure to stop at a phone box and call home to listen to the messages to make sure I wasn't about to drive all the way back to Dulverton only to have to go all the way back across the moors again. Of course this didn't always work but it was the best we had. The answering machine played a jingly tune while it rewound itself to play the messages and the longer the tune played the worse my day was about to get. Having been working there for a fair few months by this time, I'd already started to have nightmares about the tune on the answering machine and what it could mean. I remember one day in the midst of lambing I had been out on quite a lengthy call to Exford, one of our furthest destinations. I went to the usual phone box on the way back from the farm to see if there were any calls nearby. On very rare occasions I heard the wonderful words 'You have no new messages', but on this occasion it seemed unlikely because we'd been so busy recently. It was the middle of the afternoon on the Sunday of a weekend on call and I was all but dead on my feet, feeling like I'd been up since Friday morning. I dialled the home number, put the code in and waited. The tune started playing while the tape rewound itself. And played. And played. I exhaled a huge sigh and leaned my head against the side of the phone box as I listened. Finally the tune stopped and the machine cheerily announced, 'You have sixteen new messages.' SIXTEEN! I looked at the small scrap of paper I optimistically had clutched in my hand to jot the calls down on and realised it was futile. I hung up, traipsed to the car to get a bigger piece of paper and went back to go through the whole performance again before trying to plan the order in which to geographically and clinically triage the rest of my ruined day.

I'd been told earlier in the year that lambing time was 'a lot busier' than the rest of the year but I was totally unprepared for the workload and lack of sleep. I shouldn't really have been surprised because the bulk of our farm work involved sheep and when there are hundreds, if not thousands, of animals about to give birth in a six-week period then someone is going to have their work cut out for them – and that someone is the local vet. The work started as a steady trickle and over the next few weeks reached a horrific crescendo, which left me feeling like a zombie from some second-rate horror film. You've all heard of counting sheep to get to sleep but I started to feel like sheep were the source of eternal nightmares. There were sheep everywhere! I was drowning in a sea of fleece and placental juices. We could barely get the lambing ropes and surgical kits sterilised quickly enough to keep up with the demand and I noticed with interest that the little odd muscles in between my thumb and the rest of my hand were starting to look oddly out of proportion from holding on tightly to so many tiny slippery feet in my attempts to free lambs from their uterine hiding places.

Nights on call became a farce because I was simply out all night, and whole weekends passed by in the same way. I'd plough through the visits and finally head home after the kind of phone box experiences I've described only to find a line of trailers at the surgery with farmers who'd just decided to come down and wait for me to get back rather than bother me by leaving a message. It was an incredible experience, one which gave the Beeb a bumper crop of stories and left me with some very powerful memories.

On the subject of the Beeb, it soon became clear that the film crew was there for the fly-on-the-wall aspect of my life and wanted at all costs to avoid being what they would describe as 'self-referential'. In other words, this meant that they would not lift a finger to help when the faeces met the fan. They would, however, go out of their way to stay right on my tail and film the whole thing when something started to go unexpectedly pear-shaped.

On one particularly grey and drizzly morning, I saw a lovely farmer called Glen, who always brightened my day. He'd come to the surgery with two sheep which needed some treatment in a small trailer. I had already dealt with one and we'd swapped them over and put the first woolly madam (or Steve McQueen as she will now be known) back in the trailer. I was busily inspecting the fairly disgusting prolapsed vagina of the second sheep, which was covered in maggots, with the farmer peering over one shoulder and the camera wedged over the other, when there came a clattering noise from outside our little inspection shed and an excited half-yelp from one of the crew.

You would be totally astounded at the heights that can be scaled or leapt in a single bound by some of the most unwieldy and cumbersome-looking animals, including beef cattle, so the fact that this sheep had managed to ping itself neatly out of the trailer shouldn't have been that surprising. As we emerged from the shed I could tell that she had obviously surprised herself because she had a look about her which clearly said she now didn't know what to do with her newfound freedom. However dim-witted we assume sheep to be, her brain functioned more quickly than mine in that split second as she weighed her options of either staying in the car park and being cornered or heading straight down the narrow driveway that led from the practice and into the big wide open. And of course she picked the latter and set off towards the road.

You may remember that previously when chasing an unwilling beast I had longed for a Border collie. I now had a Border collie but sadly a rather gormless, six-month-old one with all the training and innate sheepdogginess of a rather bored goldfish. I was pondering testing Badger out for unrevealed talents and as I deliberated I recalled the moment a few days before when I had had cause to test his simplest of recall abilities. He had seen an elderly and very well-to-do lady positively stalking down the street, chin held high and wearing a beautiful cream, ankle-length coat. Badger and I had just come from a very muddy walk by the river and he spotted her a mile away and decided he just had to say hello. He'd set off with a wag of his ridiculously long tail and the youthful exuberance only a young dog can display and went haring towards her. I knew immediately what was going to happen because he hadn't quite got the hang of the four-paws-on-the-floor rule yet and I bellowed after him in utterly terrified panic. Time slowed down as he completely ignored me because he was simply so delighted to see this total stranger; about a metre away from her he launched himself gracefully into the air like a black-and-white torpedo and smeared river mud accurately and comprehensively down her entire front. Saying she wasn't happy would be like saying the *Titanic* had a spot of bother with an ice cube on its maiden voyage.

As the scene replayed itself in my head I discarded the idea of Badger for the job instantly and turned to the farmer. That was when I first noticed clearly that he used a stick and walked with a pronounced limp. Hmm. The farmer and I exchanged glances and set off after the sheep simultaneously, with the film crew in hot pursuit. Her first danger was the main road at the end of the surgery driveway. She came to the road edge, stopped, looked both ways as if checking for traffic and opted for her right, up into the village. We gamely followed and there ensued a farcical chase whereby an unfit woman and a lame farmer tried to catch a sheep in the prime of her life aided by reflexes honed to escape capture by millennia of evolution. We didn't stand a chance. After about twenty minutes we'd followed her a fair distance and found ourselves in the local campsite by the river getting more than our fair share of odd looks from holidaymakers, no doubt having their curiosity not only piqued by our shenanigans but by the fact that an entire film crew was running after us. It felt like an impossible task and I just couldn't see how we were going to get anywhere near her when she finally seemed to realise she had no other sheep for security, she didn't know where she was and probably she couldn't quite remember who she was or what she was doing there in the first place. At this point I wish I could say that, with a daring and spectacularly well-thought-out plan, I captured her with total disregard for my own safety and with heroic selflessness, but actually I was fit to collapse. The sheep gave up and the farmer limped up to her, hooked his crook-cum-walking-stick firmly round her neck and carried her back to the trailer with me wheezing along behind him. I really needed to start getting some exercise. As I found out later after years of numerous strangers saying, 'Ha ha, wasn't it funny when that sheep got away from you?', this incident stayed in the memories of the television-viewing public much longer than many of my more brilliant moments.

Aside from the occasional weird event such as dealing with an escapologist-sheep, lambing time and sheep-work in general showed me more in my early days as a vet than any other part of my job. Books can teach you many things but in vetting, just as in many other areas of life, seeing and experiencing things yourself is completely invaluable. The funny incidents stay with you but often not as strongly as the grim sights and strange cases. I hope you'll forgive me if I share a few such things with you and I hope that you share my sense of morbid fascination where these things are concerned. If not, skip forward to the next chapter!

I don't know if it is the pure scientist in me but ever since I was a child I have always loved the knowledge and understanding of all things biological, and often when biology goes wrong it is the most fascinating of all. As my interests have become honed into the skills of veterinary medicine and surgery, my fascination has grown too, and I am constantly filled with wonder at the incredible things our bodies and nature combine to achieve. Having said that, being a vet has given me a stomach of steel when it comes to animal matters that may make many squirm – but put an injured human in front of me and my stomach churns with the best of them!

My love of the weird and wonderful spills over a little too much sometimes, which is why I ask forgiveness from the outset. I remember one incident where I had removed a spectacularly large and pus-filled uterus, called a pyometra, from a very poorly bitch. Animals suffering from this condition are usually very ill and feel dreadful, and it can certainly be fatal, but equally they usually respond amazingly once the antibiotics start to work and the offending organ is removed. The uterus from this animal was so massive that I was totally convinced the owner would want to see it and marvel at it the way I had, but strangely she was not so keen when given the option and regarded me with a look of mild horror at the suggestion. Over the years I've realised that maybe not everyone shares my love of gross disease states, particularly, it seems, when the things have been removed from their own pets!

Anyway, farmers tend to be a bit more used to this sort of thing and less easily disgusted so the farm days were a great time for sharing my morbid discoveries with the not-so-lucky owners of the affected animals. By the end of lambing time I'd become very accustomed to a number of things that happened, and also with a rather sad fact of life about the economics of sheep farming at the time. With money a scarce commodity in farming, and sheep not being worth much back then, animals were sometimes brought to us just a little too late for us to be able to help. Or sometimes a lot too late. This wasn't always anyone's fault: with the best will in the world some sheep don't get spotted trying to lamb until they've been at it for hours or even days, and usually by then the lamb is not only dead but is starting to rot. I won't forget the first time a whole front leg came off when I was pulling a lamb out in a hurry. Fear not: at this stage a lamb is a long way past living and the best thing we can do is get the toxic carcass out to try to save the mother. The fact is that bits falling off were always preceded by a very characteristic smell of rotting lambswool and one that I soon came to recognise instantly.

One of these was a case of *schistosomus reflexus*. When the ewe in question came to me this time there was no mistaking the smell and I knew the job was going to be a grim one of salvaging the mother rather than a joyful presentation of a gorgeous lamb to the udder after all our efforts. As a great veterinary obstetrics teacher who taught a friend of mine in Edinburgh always says, the three linchpins of obstetrics (and any dealings with the ladies, he suggests) are sensitivity, patience and plenty of lubrication (a wise man indeed), and the last of these three is certainly a must for these cases which have gone on too long. As I felt gently inside I quickly realised I could feel bones instead of skin and was sure I was feeling my first schistosome lamb. These animals, through a quirk of conception, form completely inside out.

When any mammal is formed in the uterus it is like a Smarties tube to all intents and purposes. It starts at one seam, which represents the spine if you like, and grows round to meet in the middle of the abdomen and chest, enclosing all the soft, squidgy bits in the middle. In a schistosome all the limbs and organs form as normal but the tube goes the wrong way, so the organs and the spine end up on the outside and in our analogy you drop your Smarties all over the floor. These poor creatures never survive and so this became a horrible job of trying to remove the dead lamb, but at least we saved the mother to try again next year. Such cases are pretty rare and could easily stay in the confines of a textbook through most vets' lives. Although it may sound morbid, my fascination with the incredible process of making new life meant that, although very sad, this was a case that I'll always be grateful I saw.

The other really odd abnormality I saw belonged to a farmer called Peter, one of my favourite clients. Many farmers are really adept at lambing their own sheep and have way more experience than a young graduate like I was then. Peter was one of these farmers, and when he needed help it was always for a genuine reason. He'd phoned one day and asked if he could bring a ewe in to be lambed, which was pretty unusual for him, and described something 'weird hanging out the back end'. I was certainly intrigued and the BBC had no doubt they were going to follow this one.

When he arrived we got the sheep out and into the examination shed and it became very clear that he wasn't joking. There was what appeared at first glance to be a normally coloured and fleeced part of a lamb protruding from the sheep and she was gamely straining away trying to shift the thing. The problem was that the only bits of a lamb that can get this far are the nose, the tail or a combination of legs and feet and what I could see didn't look like any of those things. I tried to feel round the edges of it but the whole birth canal was full of this odd thing. It quickly became obvious that the only option was going to be a Caesarean section to get the lamb out and I wasn't at all sure what was going on.

Once the sheep had had a local anaesthetic along her flank and was clean and as sterile as we could hope for I made my incision. As I felt into the abdomen to bring the uterus up to the wound to get the lamb out I realised I was going to need a bigger hole. The whole abdomen seemed to be taken up with this uterus. I felt along it and the monster size of the lamb became evident. The whole thing felt like a floppy balloon of water the likes of which I'd never experienced. I extended the incision and found that the whole lamb was just a giant bag of skin and fluid, the legs were tree trunks of water under the wool and the thing as a whole was absolutely massive. It was what is called a hydrops, a bloated and malformed creature full of fluid. I finally managed to get it out and tried to carefully place it on the floor of the shed as gently as I could but it weighed a ton and kind of flopped onto the ground with an awful squishing sound. The lamb had no chance of survival. It seemed that it was going to be a sad and unfruitful day for Peter and I turned back to the ewe to concentrate on getting her stitched up and on the road to recovery as soon as possible.

As I was about to close the uterus I remembered one of the lessons that had been drummed into us repeatedly as students;

you ALWAYS check for another offspring, even in cows and horses which usually only have one and even when it seems impossible. I mentally mocked myself for thinking this because the monster lamb had filled up the whole sheep, let alone the uterus, but they tell us these things for a reason and it was ingrained, so I went to have a cursory feel around. I felt sure this was a futile formality, but I found to my complete and utter astonishment that there was a tiny sibling to this monster tucked away in the darkest recesses of its mother. Against all the odds this tiny lamb was otherwise normal and alive and I called to Peter to take it from me and to try to get it going while I saw to its mum.

The lamb was very weak and small and it didn't start breathing as we had hoped. I was asking for updates as I frantically sutured the large incisions in all the layers of its mother's muscle and skin. Finally, I went outside to Peter's Land Rover, where he had the tiny lamb huddled into the footwell, bundled up for warmth. I gave the lamb some drops of a breathing stimulant under its tongue. It gradually started to breathe a little more deeply and finally let out the wonderful little bleat that we'd all been waiting to hear. Reunited with its mum it had the best chance of survival as she cleaned and nestled and cajoled it to life, all the time making the most endearing little noises of encouragement. It was a fantastic and unexpected end to what had seemed such a sad and grotesque case and is a shining example of what makes the job so brilliant.

I said at the start of this chapter that lambing taught me more in a short space of time than any other period I can recall, and it wasn't only about the oddities that are produced when nature gets it wrong. It's a sad fact of life as a farm vet that you quickly become accustomed to death and the fact that reproduction isn't always a time of celebration, but I also learnt in those six weeks that, no matter how hardened you think you are to life and death, you can never be prepared for some things. There is one memory that I would rather shed from my brain but I know will stay with me forever. I'd been pottering about tending to some in-patients in the lambing shed at the surgery when I heard a truck pull up outside. I went out to investigate and there was a farmer there I'd not met before. He introduced himself and apologised for not having phoned beforehand but asked me to look at three sheep he had in the back of his pickup. The sheep were all unrestrained and could have easily escaped but they were going nowhere, that much was obvious immediately.

I examined each in turn and all had similar injuries and all were in a numb state of shock. Sheep are surprisingly well protected by their thick fleeces but there are a few places like the belly and the neck which are vulnerable to attack by predators and whatever had attacked these sheep had known just where to go. All three had varying degrees of rips and tears to the softest, most vulnerable places. Two of them I had to euthanise immediately because of bowel damage but the third I managed to save, probably only because the damage was so mild compared to the other two. I'd never seen anything like it and asked the farmer if he knew what had happened. He'd had a grim and ashen face since he arrived but if anything the colour seemed to drain away even more as he exhaled a sad and furious sigh and said that his neighbour's three dogs had broken into the field and run amok. I was horrified for this poor man and his animals but unbeknown to me I'd only seen the tip of the iceberg. It was at this point that he showed me what I had paid no heed to at all as I'd examined the three injured sheep; the tarpaulin-covered cargo of the rest of the truck.

He walked to the side of his truck with a defeated air, got hold of a corner of the blue plastic tarpaulin and pulled it back in one sweeping gesture like a magician about to say a triumphant 'ta-da!' But there was nothing magical about what was laid bare. The whole pickup was full of dead sheep. There was a pile of what must have been twenty or more thrown higgledy-piggledy in the back. They had all been due to give birth in the next few weeks and they lay there, throats and bowels torn asunder in one of the most gruesome and soul-destroying sights I have ever seen. We both stood and simply stared. He was clearly grief-stricken and I was stunned. After a long silence I asked quietly, 'What will you do about the dogs?'

There was barely a second's hesitation before his answer knocked the air out of me as much as the sight of his slain sheep had. 'I've shot all three of them dead.'

I am an animal lover above most other things and the senseless tragedy of this will never leave me. I was heartbroken about the dogs but, having seen what they'd done, I knew he'd had no choice, especially when he told me that, unbelievably, this was the second time his neighbours had let it happen. I'm sorry to tell such a horrible tale but these things need to be heard. We somehow hold pets more highly than their meat-providing counterparts. Some see sheep as being stupid or somehow worthless, but those sheep had suffered terribly and he knew that many of the others that had survived would lose their lambs or even die later themselves through shock. Whatever your view of sheep versus dog, he'd done the only thing he could do to save his animals.

Although this tragic story is absolutely awful, and many of the events I've described in this chapter are strange and sad, that doesn't tell the whole truth of lambing time. I suppose it's simply human nature to remember the weird, wonderful and grim before the routine, everyday and positive things in life. What a funny species we are. Lambing time was body-breakingly hectic but it is still one of my fondest times to remember in many ways. I can't tell you often enough how magical birth is and what a privilege it is to be involved in it in all its varying glories. As vets, the sad fact is that by the nature of our job it is only the problem births we see, not the normal ones, so inevitably some of these are not going to end well. But for every rotting, awful thing I saw that spring there were countless times where these beautiful little creatures were just a bit eager to get out and things had simply gone a bit skew-whiff, so to speak. Mostly they'd just need straightening out and pulling out. Often there'd be two or three eager young things trying to get out all at the same time and you'd just need to wag a finger at them and say 'tut tut' and then put them into an orderly queue to take them out one by one. It didn't matter how tired I was or how saddened by something I'd seen: there was nothing in the world that could keep a smile from my face when the next lamb to appear would take a breath, shake the worst of the goo from itself and call to its mother for the first time. That's solid gold, and those memories are some that I treasure the most from my time working on Exmoor.

Coming, as I do, from a pacifist upbringing by 'hippy' parents in the Medway Towns in Kent, the abundance of guns in the area in which I worked was a bit of a shock to me, and the shooting of the dogs made a huge impact. When I was seeing practice I'd had my first encounter with firearms and they are incredibly scary things. I'd seen a vet shoot a cow and, as naive as it might sound, the noise and the violent suddenness of the death were absolutely startling. I use the words 'violent' and 'startling' but in fact shooting, when done the right way, is a very humane way indeed of killing an animal. Everyone has their own views on gun laws and whether guns kill people or people kill people, but I firmly believe that people certainly wouldn't kill as many other people if they didn't have guns to hand! Firearms are surely accidents waiting to happen.

We had a wonderfully eccentric client in Exmoor called Roger, who roped his cattle like a cowboy and was a fantastic character. Like many farmers he had several shotguns which, when combined with his eccentricity, was always a bit of a worry, but when the inevitable accident did happen, it was thankfully more funny than anything else. Roger had a beautiful old farmhouse with large drawing rooms, which were immaculately decorated and festooned with a wonderful array of rural ornaments pertaining to the age-old pursuits of shooting and fishing. Whenever I was at the farm I always felt like I should be deloused or at least hosed down before being allowed to enter the inner sanctum of the place. It was worlds away from the muck and filth that covered the outside of most of the other farms I encountered.

Being the owner of such an immaculate household, Roger was taken aback one day to see that a dirty great crow had flown down the chimney into one of his beautiful show-home type rooms. It had become trapped and was sitting covered in soot on the hearth, looking a little dazed. I don't know what the normal response to this situation would be, but it might involve creeping away to get a sheet or blanket to throw over the bird in order to capture it. For some reason Roger opted to run from the room, grab the nearest shotgun and try to kill the bird before it could cause any damage. An airgun pellet from a quiet and non-threatening distance might have been more appropriate but, as Roger careered angrily into the room like Elmer Fudd after Bugs Bunny, the terrified bird took flight and started spraying soot all round the room, flapping willy-nilly among the prized ornaments. All would not have been lost for most normal folk, who might have admitted defeat and waited for the bird to tire itself out, but, not being one to be defeated by such a pesky critter, Roger let fly with a volley of hurriedly aimed shots as the bird winged its way round the room. I've got no idea whether he actually managed to shoot the thing but, judging by his exasperated look as he told me the story, I'm guessing the damage to the room from the shotgun was pretty considerable. It was all I could do not to burst out laughing as I tried to retain the serious and sympathetic look on my face.

Eventually, working in a large-animal practice I inevitably found myself in a situation where I needed to handle a gun and actually shoot an animal myself, and that happened to be in lambing time too. I'd had a sheep brought in which was bleeding uncontrollably from a huge ruptured artery in its womb. By the time the ewe got to the surgery she had lost too much blood for me to save her, but she was in the process of lambing so my best option was to shoot her and immediately remove the lambs in the hope of saving them. Shooting was the best option because, if I'd used the drugs we use for small animals, the lambs would have received the drug straight across the placenta and been killed along with their mother.

As it turned out, Mr Elliot had the gun because he'd needed it on another call so I rang him and he rushed to the surgery with it. Because I'd never used a gun before, and because Mr Elliot had to actually bring it in, I was desperately hoping that he would just do it for me because I was really nervous about handling it. The BBC had been filming the whole case too so there was an added pressure. As Mr Elliot arrived I followed him into the surgery and implored him to shoot the sheep, but to my immense disappointment he said no. I don't know whether it was because he thought I should get on and learn or just because he had always been reluctant to be filmed, but I remember wanting to beg and plead with him to do it despite knowing there was no point. It was clear from his tone that I was on my own. I took the gun box, shut myself in the lambing shed and told the reluctant crew to leave. It felt dangerous enough going into what was essentially a concrete-lined box with a pistol without trying to cram more bodies in there to get in the way of the bullet if anything went wrong.

The gun was a one-shot pistol with no safety catch so once it was loaded it was lethal. I was totally petrified and felt like a dangerous psychopath. As soon as I'd clicked the bullet into place I became convinced that a catastrophe would happen. I would be killed by a ricochet, the gun would go off accidentally or I'd have a moment of madness and just shoot anything except the sheep. I wanted rid of the situation as quickly as I could so I stepped to the doomed animal, took aim and fired.

I'm sure I must have shut my eyes as I pulled the trigger, which isn't exactly what a highly trained sniper would do, but the job was done and I hadn't been got by a stray ricochet or any of the other irrational things I'd expected to happen. As quickly as I could I cut into the sheep's abdomen and pulled the lamb out but despite all our efforts I was just too late. It was another of the many experiences on the steep learning curve of my first job that my mum would definitely call 'character-building'. It also became one more in a string of times that Mr Elliot and I had locked horns and it seemed I was never on the winning end of these encounters. The whole gun episode became another nail in the coffin of any resolve I had to stay. A few months later the final nail went in.

At the time I worked at the practice all the sterilisation of surgical instruments was done using chemicals. Basically this involved the instruments being washed and then placed in a bucket full of pretty toxic stuff that killed every bug known to man. Once sterile, the instruments were removed, left to dry and placed in polythene bags until they were used. It was a pretty antiquated way of doing the job and I'd been badgering the partners for an autoclave. This is like a powerful, high-temperature pressure cooker, which very effectively does the job of sterilisation and also removes any possibility of contamination by handling the instruments afterwards because they are sealed in sterile bags. Eventually Martin and I had worn Mr Elliot down and he'd agreed that I could source a second-hand machine. I'd found one for a really reasonable price and showed Mary and Bretia how to use it and how to bag up the instruments using a special tape which changed colour when the instruments were sterile. I was very happy.

Joe and I went away camping for a week about a month after we'd bought the autoclave and when I got back it took me a while to put my finger on what was missing from the worktop in the practice. A few minutes later it struck me that the missing item was my beloved autoclave, so I went looking for the specially designed rolls of bag material and sterility-indicating tape. It was all gone. I asked Mary where it was, wondering if the second-hand machine had malfunctioned.

'Mr Elliot sent it back,' she said quietly, averting her eyes because she knew how disappointed I'd be. I don't think I said anything in return, but I was livid and went home later that night fuming. It might be a small thing to many people but it left me feeling like my surgery, and therefore my integrity as a vet, was being compromised, and I'd just got to the stage that I felt I couldn't put up with it any more. I'd also started to realise over the course of the year that I really wanted to specialise in small animals. I loved the farm work in many ways and the farmers particularly, but I found the economics of farm practice very frustrating. As a vet you want to do everything in your power to alleviate suffering and cure disease, but economics often meant that farm animals were put to sleep because the money simply wasn't there to treat them or nurse them back to health. This isn't the farmers' fault, it's just the reality of the world. I'd also started to feel that Dulverton was just a bit too small to occupy the social needs of a twenty-something and all these things heaped together meant it was time to go. But go where?

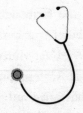

Chapter 5

Mirror, mirror, on the wall...

Phil, one of my friends from university, is a consultant ophthalmologist now but I'm sure he's wasted in that job. With his savage wit and dry delivery he probably should have made his career as a stand-up comedian. Phil had been working in Cheltenham for some time and had told me it was a great place and that I should move there. Quite by one of life's total coincidences, a surfing friend of Joe's, who he'd met on holiday on the other side of the world, also lived there and said the same thing. I started scanning the good old *Veterinary Record* and in one of those seemingly random twists of fate there was a job being advertised in Cheltenham that was a decent increase in salary but, most appealingly, had a one in eight rota. It sounded like heaven compared to my one in three. I was sold. I wanted the job there and then and suddenly I couldn't wait to be gone and realised how much I was ready to move on. I plucked up the last of my courage and went to see Mr Elliot in his office for the final time. It was only a week or two after the autoclave had gone back and he didn't seem surprised at all when I told him I was handing in my notice. Rash young things that we were, we decided we were going to move before I even found out whether I had the job in Cheltenham. There were a few jobs going in the surrounding area and I was pretty sure I'd get one of them even if it wasn't the one I'd set my heart on. Exciting times were afoot.

It was during my last few weeks at the practice that the latest series of *Vets In Practice* was aired and the end of the series featured the fact that I was moving on. I was away visiting some friends in Bristol when the programme about my leaving came on, and I was totally mortified. I watched in horror as I saw myself being interviewed and saying some pretty uncomplimentary things about the place. I must have been caught on a particularly off day and I think I had started to call the village Dulltown instead of Dulverton, and I couldn't believe it was being shown before I'd escaped. I was so embarrassed. I've always hated confrontational situations and I would never knowingly upset anyone but I'd said these terrible things and then I had to go back there! I felt like I should do a stealth mission to move out but the cat was out of the bag and I had to endure a few fairly black looks and some pointed comments before I finally left. So, in hindsight, to all the good folks of Dulverton – sorry! I did have some fun times but it was just the right time to move on.

I managed to badger the owner of the practice in Cheltenham into giving me the job and had had a guided tour when I went for the interview. The practice had recently expanded by opening a branch on the other side of town and Barry, the owner, was in the midst of doing much of the refurbishment of the new branch himself when I applied for the job. I've found over the years that many veterinary interviews tend to be quite informal: a chat and a look round with questions from both parties and then a general feeling about whether you like each other. There aren't clinical questions or tests, at least in the ones I've been to, I suppose because it is assumed that vets of any certain length of experience should be capable of doing what's expected. Barry and I would alternate between the two branches on a daily basis, often meeting at the newer branch which had the more up-to-date facilities to do the bulk of the ops together. This was good for me because I still got continuity with clients and had to stand on my own two feet to make decisions, but I also got help with operations I'd never done before. I was looking forward to getting stuck into a lot more small-animal surgery than we'd done in Dulverton.

Before any of this could happen Joe and I were faced with the daunting tasks of finding somewhere to rent that would allow us and our five animals to move in, and also finding Joe somewhere to work. In the meantime we were homeless, so we packed Pan and Badger off to my parents' house in Kent and some good friends of the family agreed to board our motley crew of cats while we sorted ourselves out. By the time six weeks had passed we'd been sleeping on the floor of a friend's house in Bristol and commuting to Cheltenham, Badger and

Pan had totally devastated mum and dad's garden and seemed to be trying to dig their way to the other side of the world, and everyone involved was very relieved indeed when we found a lovely bungalow to rent that accepted pets. We gathered our belongings and our misbehaving dogs, and made the big step of moving in together for the first time to start our new life in Cheltenham.

Once we'd had a week or so to get organised it was time to get the cats back and complete the family circle. By this time the cats were all about a year to eighteen months old and had developed very distinct characteristics and personalities. Charlie had his beautiful biscuit-coloured coat, his missing back leg and his incessant and sometimes *very* annoying yowling. If Nigel were a posh new hybrid, he would be a Labrasloth. His combination of appetite and laziness was strangely causing his head to shrink (admittedly this is an unforgivable way of saying that he is ever so slightly overweight) but it was Brian who had developed the lion's share of quirkiness. I know you're not allowed favourites but Brian has always been my favourite cat. He paddles in the water bowl before having a drink although I have no idea why and seems to have the curious notion that he is in fact a dog. At a very young age he decided that Badger was his favourite thing in the world and then attached himself surgically to Badger's side, including when out for a walk near the house. When Badger settles down to sleep, Brian is there like a shot, curling up in amongst his legs and kneading him like he's frantically making bread. Badger tries to tolerate this as much as possible but eventually tires of it and retaliates by gently placing the whole of Brian's head in his mouth and giving it a gentle squeeze. Brian gets the message and stops bread making and looks steadfastly in the other direction as if butter wouldn't melt in his mouth and waits for a few seconds. As soon as Badger lets go and settles back down, Brian practically gives a nonchalant whistle, tries to look innocent and starts all over again, happily purring and clawing the poor long-suffering Badger in the side. He always makes me think of the line from *Monty Python's Life of Brian*; 'He's *not* the Messiah. He's a very naughty boy!'

The bungalow we'd rented was in a fairly upmarket part of town near the surgery. It had a slightly odd location in that it sat in a kind of open space which formed the access to the rear of some lovely regency houses but didn't really have any obvious neighbours. About a month after we moved Joe had found a great job which was only part-time so he was often home when I got in from work. One evening I arrived back and wandered into the kitchen to get the obligatory post-work glass of wine. On the kitchen floor was a very beautifully made glove puppet of the children's character Sooty. I could hear Joe was in the bath and I called out, 'Where did the Sooty puppet come from?' assuming Joe had picked it up somewhere for the boys to play with. After a couple of seconds' delay he murmured from deep in a surf magazine, 'What puppet?' with all the interest of the dead. I shrugged to myself and thought nothing more of it, although in hindsight, it's odd that I didn't question more strongly how it came to be in the house.

The next day when I went into the kitchen there was a plush, expensive-looking owl puppet laid tenderly on the kitchen floor. Now my interest was really piqued. I leaned against the worktop and stared inquisitively at the latest arrival. Where had it come from? Was Joe turning into a weird kleptomaniac or breaking into houses in some somnambulatory trance? I picked up the toy and put it next to Sooty on the worktop. Things got very surreal on the third day when I found Sweep. Going to the kitchen was starting to be like Christmas. I couldn't wait to see what had arrived overnight. I'd just picked Sweep up and was pondering doing my own puppet show when I heard the distinctive clatter of the cat flap. I instinctively turned at the noise and that was when all became clear. Brian was halfway through the flap with a brilliantly coloured sock puppet, the type my mum used to make when we were kids.

Brian saw me the minute he got his head through the flap with his special prize. He froze instantly, one foot in and one foot out, and stared intently at a spot in his middle distance. At the same time I had subconsciously frozen too and so there we were, locked in a bizarre Mexican stand-off. It was evident that Brian believed that if he stayed completely still I couldn't possibly see him. The fact that he is bright ginger, quite large and was dragging a bright blue sock with gaudy yellow eyes stitched onto it seemed to have escaped him. After what seemed like an eternity but was probably about two seconds he obviously got bored, realised it was a fair cop and hauled the rest of the sock into the kitchen, dumped it unceremoniously on the floor and sauntered off as if it was the most natural thing in the world for one of the planet's most finely honed hunters to bring toys made out of hosiery proudly home.

The next few days brought two more puppets and a large pair of furry blue men's slippers. The most impressive thing about the latter was that he had obviously had to make two trips to make sure he brought the pair. By now we were in a bit of a quandary. Somewhere nearby a small child was almost certainly being badly scolded, if not beaten, not only for losing so many lovely toys but probably for appearing to lie about it too. But we had the fear that by now we'd left it too long. How could we own up that our cat was a cat-burglar? What if the owners of the toys wanted us to get rid of him or make monetary reparations for the soggy and rather dirty slippers? Added to which we had no real neighbours, so how far afield and in what direction should we go? I confess, after all these years, that we never tried to find out. If, in the late nineties, you were about six and living near The Park in Cheltenham and you've been mentally scarred by the gradual disappearance of your favourite toys and your dad's slippers, I apologise unreservedly. It wasn't me, it was the cat! The trickle of gifts stopped as suddenly as it had started and I was left wondering if there was some way I could train Brian to get better bounty next time round.

The job in Cheltenham had a lot of things going for it and I was glad we'd made the move. We had some great nurses and I'd made some very good friends. Having come from a job where we had no qualified nurses at all and very little equipment it was brilliant to have qualified help and to be able to start indulging my passion for small-animal surgery. I was still young and pretty green and I was loving the new challenges that the job brought with it. We worked long days and although the rota was fantastic compared to one in three we were on call for four practices at a time so the on-call was usually pretty frantic. But I was used to that and was still trying to break the habit of sleeping fully clothed when I was on duty.

By the time we moved to Cheltenham *Vets in Practice* had gained hugely in popularity and was regularly getting around eight million viewers, which is quite incredible these days. I found that I'd become a kind of pseudo-celebrity, caught in an odd limbo, with a very normal working life interspersed with the occasional plunge into an entirely different world of exciting celebrity adventures. But that's not to say I haven't made some bad choices when it comes to such 'celebrity' opportunities.

I'd already done a few appearances on things like *Richard and Judy* but then I got asked if I'd like to go on a programme called *Style Challenge*. This was a makeover show on during the morning, which I'd heard of but not seen. It sounded like fun and they wanted to make a 'celebrity' edition of it featuring me and Trude. Although I knew Trude pretty well from going through vet school together, we'd moved in different circles during the five years so we weren't close friends, but when I heard she'd accepted the offer it bolstered my confidence that I should too. Safety in numbers, right? The fact that she was the blonde Norwegian bombshell from the series should have alerted me to the possibility that I might not come off looking great because it was like asking Ann Widdecombe to go up against Pamela Anderson in a swimsuit competition, but I was young and, as it turned out, monumentally stupid, so I said yes.

I'd had the same hairstyle for ever and a day and I've never had the money or the style to be fashionable, so in my head I conjured up images of being turned from an ugly duckling into an amazingly beautiful superstar. The show was hosted by Oz Clarke of wine fame and they had top hairdressers and stylists to do the makeover. I was asked if there was an event coming up they could concentrate on making me over for. I had a friend's wedding in a few months so I suggested that and they were happy to give it a try. When asked about things I didn't want I said I didn't mind entering into the spirit of it as long as they didn't expect me to wear heels and I didn't want to be given a hat just because it was a wedding.

The big day arrived and I was pretty excited. Trevor Sorbie was my 'hairdresser to the stars' and he came into the dressing room beforehand and asked me what I thought I'd like. I'm cringing just thinking about this but at the time I was a big fan of Meg Ryan and I'd seen a film called *French Kiss* in which she looked beautiful and short-haired. Obviously now I realise that she looks that way because she's an actress with an entourage of hair and make-up people and because she is actually beautiful, but I had high hopes and Trevor looked very happy that for once he was going to be allowed to actually cut someone's hair off instead of just styling it.

The idea was that Trude and I would have our hair and make-up done in front of the audience and then be taken off to get togged up in our lovely new clothes and then have to stand in front of a mirror and have our new look revealed to us in front of the audience. I can feel a cold sweat starting with the memory. I sat on the stage and Trevor set about my do like Edward Scissorhands on speed and the make-up artist set to work. I was then taken off backstage to be dressed. This was done blindfolded so you didn't know what you looked like. I could see a strip of light at the bottom of the blindfold and I knew I had what looked like quite a slinky black dress on, which pleased me because my figure wasn't too bad at the time. Then of course to ruin it all they put an awful, typically 'wedding', pastel-blue jacket on me and, contrary to everything I'd said, bloody great high heels and a *hat*! Being the meek and timid creature that I was, I didn't dare say anything so I then had to wait for my signal and parade down the catwalk in front of the cameras and the audience in one of the most awkward moments of my life. Awkward partly because I'm pretty shy in many respects and was quite embarrassed, and also because I told them not to put me in heels for a very good reason. I walk like a man in heels, and I don't mean an accomplished transvestite drag queen, I mean your average man in the street given a pair of four-inch heels and a voucher for a leg wax!

The signal came and I teetered out to rapturous and obligatory applause from the crowd and headed for the God-awful moment at the mirror. They swung it round and I sort of convulsed in this faux gratitude for how amazing I looked when in fact I was gawking in horror and convulsing with the early stages of post-traumatic stress at the fact that, instead of looking like Meg Ryan at the Oscars, I looked like Ian Beale from *EastEnders* dressed as someone from *Dallas* in the eighties. I have a strict rule in life that you must never have regrets and should instead embrace all experiences as learning opportunities, but this was going to test that rule to the limit. If ever I wanted to shrivel up and disappear, this was it. Of course then Trude was revealed and looked like a Scandinavian goddess, because she is, which only heightened the fact that I looked like an extremely awkward, gender-confused boy.

In the days that followed I could only console myself with the fact that the programme was on mid-morning, so no one would ever see it, but the coming weeks proved to my endless horror and shame how many of my clients watched daytime television, because it seemed that every second person through the door had seen the damn thing. I fake-smiled my way through weeks of consultations, having to repeatedly re-live the awful 'big mirror moment', and waited for the fallout to settle down and go away forever. I'd almost got over it when months and months later I got an email from a friend saying with glee that it was going to be repeated on prime time because it was a celebrity special. It seemed that the fact that I am and always will be, even with professional help, style-challenged rather than a *Style Challenge* would haunt me to the end of time.

As I have said, the celebrity aspects of my odd life back then were very few and far between and the majority of my time was spent at work doing the job I'd strived my whole life to do. Switching from a very mixed, country job to just small-animal work in a town brought with it some changes in clientele, which took a little getting used to. We had a frantically busy diary with ten-minute appointments, which often ended up being squeezed into five minutes as extras got wedged in wherever they would fit. Gone were the days of my leisurely farm visits and open surgeries. Now it was go, go, go and I often felt like I barely had time to catch my breath between patients.

I also had to get used to the fact that I wasn't dealing with salt-of-the-earth farmer types any more. Now my clients were all pet owners, all madly in love with their animals and, occasionally, just mad! The array of people you encounter as a vet is incredible. It's an obvious thing to say but many would-be vets fall by the wayside because they just wanted to work with animals and fail to realise that the animals always come in with a human: dealing with owners can be way trickier than dealing with a savage hamster. I must say that we had loads of wonderful clients but I did have to get used to the way small-animal clients describe what's wrong with their animals. Farmers are used to talking about genitals, faeces and bodily functions but the general public, I was about to learn, are a little more bashful or sometimes just confused.

A classic area of confusion is the removal of sex organs. This is an incredibly routine thing that virtually all vets recommend. It stops animals wandering, fighting and spreading diseases. It also prevents or alleviates all sorts of life-threatening and horrible diseases in old age. The word 'neutering' is perfectly acceptable for both sexes; castration refers solely to males and spaying solely to females. It's not difficult when you know but we get some wonderful variations. It's very difficult not to chuckle when someone asks you to 'splay' or 'spray' their beloved pet. It conjures up all sorts of mental images of what we might do to it. When working in Cheltenham I had one client who wanted to book their bitch in to be 'spaded'. I pondered whether the client was asking for a novel and savage form of euthanasia and wanted me to take the dog out the back and clout the poor hound with a shovel, which is pretty much what popped into my head when I heard the request. On the subject of euthanasia, you also have to be very careful indeed when people ask to have their animals 'put to sleep', because quite often they mean 'anaesthetised' and some very unfortunate things have happened to vets over the years when they've taken the owners at their word. Thankfully, communication hasn't let me down yet.

Bodily functions and bits of anatomy can also be difficult to decipher. A very well-to-do client in Dulverton had started to alert me to this whenever she described her little Yorkie's problems with its 'shooies'. It took nearly a whole consultation for me to figure out that she meant his faeces and not some sort of footwear for pampered pooches I didn't know about. Business, mess, dirt, number twos, big jobs: the list is endless when it comes to the ways people try to avoid saying faeces or poo. Genitals seem to present an even bigger challenge to our stiff-upper-lipped nation. The first time I was told that a little lapdog wouldn't leave her tuppence alone I was at a loss, and calling a penis a tail is really asking for trouble sooner or later! The fact is that as a vet or a doctor you have to get used to this weird and wonderful array of colloquial ways to avoid saying words that schoolchildren love to say as often as possible.

A director I filmed with once was involved with a countrywide BBC drive to look at regional accents and embrace and celebrate our differences. We were in the car one day and he took a phone call from a woman he wanted to interview and I heard this brilliant story on the speakerphone. This woman's job was to teach young, foreign doctors all the ways that people describe genitals and bodily problems to their GPs. It's something I'd never have thought of but if the public can't tell a vet about their pet's problems then how on earth do we expect them to use scientific terminology about their own bits and bobs? She told us that she'd had one doctor who had seen a woman who had a certain problem 'down below' and the doctor wanted to refer her, straight away that week, to a gynaecologist. The patient had looked very shy and explained that she definitely couldn't go that week because she 'had her friend with her'. The doctor told her that was no problem at all and he was sure the specialist wouldn't mind if she took her friend with her. What he had spectacularly failed to realise is that she meant that she couldn't go that week because she was having her period!

Working in a profession that deals with incredibly strong emotions and people's fears for their pets can also test your mental strength. In a job where you need to be serious so very much of the time it can be difficult to keep your mind focussed and on 'the act' when some of these strange things come out of clients' mouths. I may be accused of being immature but some situations which immerse you in a world of possible innuendo do make it very difficult not to 'corpse' like a comedic actor trying his best to keep a straight face.

During my time at this practice in Cheltenham, I had a lovely client whose cat had to come in fairly frequently because of urinary tract problems. The first time I saw this woman she reminded me of Les Dawson's large female character, hoicking her boobs firmly into position with a well-practised forearm nudge. On her first visit she heaved a huge wicker cat basket onto the table and let the enormous cat out to wander round and get used to her surroundings. She was a beautiful big ginger cat and was remarkably unfazed about being at the vet's – a thing that terrifies many an animal. Before we got down to the nitty-gritty of the actual medical problem, the owner and I were chatting about Poppy the cat by way of getting to know each other. After a minute or two, and with a very serious expression, she gave the cat an absent-minded fondle of the ears and took a deep sigh before telling me that she was having 'awful trouble with the neighbour's cat using her pussy door'. The professional in me should have taken this in my stride as a perfectly valid concern of many owners, but the sometimes uncontrollable smutty schoolchild in me decided to take it the wrong way and then I just couldn't stop thinking about the phrase 'pussy door'. I had to stroke the cat for about two full minutes before I could trust myself to speak without tears streaming down my face.

'These things are sent to try us' is a phrase often used by my mum as I was growing up, and the early years of my career as a vet were, if not exactly trying, certainly eye-poppingly varied. Getting used to the human angle of vetting wasn't going to be as easy as it might have seemed and it was in our first summer in Cheltenham that I had my first human emergency – one that highlighted some more of my inadequacies.

It was first thing Monday morning and the small waiting room was already packed. As you know by now, mornings are not my best time of day and I was groggily working my way through the second case. The practice I worked in wasn't computerised so in between clients I would go to reception with the handwritten notes on the client's card so that the nurses could make up the bill. I'd take the next card in line and call the client in. It was an absolutely scorching day and we had fans going and all the doors wide open but the room was still stifling. I was just looking at the card to see who to call when there was a loud clatter followed by a very worried, strangled noise from one of the people waiting. I looked up and the client was simply pointing, unspeaking and mouth open, to the other side of the waiting room where the clatter had come from. My gaze followed the rigid finger and, to my horror, it appeared that one of my clients had died in the opposite corner. The clatter had been the noise of the heavy plastic cat carrier, cat included, being dropped onto the floor as the man had slumped into his chair, head hanging down on his chest.

There were a distinct few seconds where I froze, staring in disbelief and totally unsure of what to do next. Eventually my morning fog disappeared in a blur of adrenalin and I raced over to the startlingly bluish-purple man. It was at this point that I realised I didn't have the faintest idea what to do. I was just feeling for a pulse on his clammy neck when someone who clearly had more inkling about humans than I had said we should lay him on the floor and put his legs in the air. However, before we could slide him off his chair the bluish-purple colour literally disappeared in a wave that travelled up from his boots to the crown of his head; as he changed to grey and then to pink, like a large prawn being cooked, he magically came back to life. I imagine from the bewildered look on his face that he was as shocked to see all of us staring at him with terrified looks on our faces as we were to have witnessed his apparent near death. He flushed with embarrassment, picked his cat up and said he must have fainted from the heat. By this time we'd called an ambulance and when we rang them back they said that because he'd lost consciousness they'd have to come anyway. The poor man was mortified to be causing so much commotion and was insisting that he was fine, but we couldn't argue with the emergency services so we sat him in the fresh air outside the door, which probably made even more of a spectacle of him, and got on with morning surgery. I realised with startling clarity that I really needed to do a human first aid course because the emergency automatic pilot I had been so proud of in the past was clearly set on animals only.

Despite all these oddities and ups and downs I soon realised that I'd survived the first few months in this new and exciting world of small-animal work and was actually really enjoying myself. It seemed like now would be as good a time as any for my next big step.

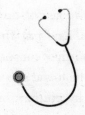

Chapter 6

Brian strikes again

So it was that eventually the time came when, having survived living together in rented accommodation, Joe and I decided to get ourselves onto the property ladder. Not long after we started looking we were extremely lucky to have an offer accepted on a gorgeous end-terrace house in Cheltenham with lots of stripped floorboards and a beautiful big stone fireplace to keep the pyromaniac in me happy. I think I've always been really lucky with how my animals have coped with moving house and they didn't let me down this time either. Our happy little band seemed to be content as long as we were all together and it didn't matter where that was. We had virtually no furniture but our first night in the new house was full of excitement and the fact that we had to sleep on a futon mattress on the floor just made it all the more romantic somehow.

We gradually started to accumulate things to sleep on and sit on and did bits and pieces of DIY to put our stamp on the place. We'd been there about a month when the next pair of slippers arrived. I was pretty used to getting up to find a multitude of elastic bands in the house, kindly and lovingly brought home by Brian, the catcher of all things inanimate. It had taken me a while to figure out why he found so many but then I realised that they were discarded by postmen once they'd unwrapped bundles of banded mail. Not very environmentally friendly if you ask me, but luckily I had a cat who was on the case of tidying up the planet single-pawedly. Elastic bands and a few half-desiccated frogs were all we'd had since the puppet fiasco of the previous year so I wasn't expecting to see the slippers, and almost did Brian the injustice of thinking he'd got sloppy and only brought one. The one I'd seen was in the kitchen near the cat flap. This time it was another large man's slipper but not furry; this one was your classic Marks and Spencer quilted tartan. Brian was sitting nearby, lazily inspecting one of his paws and glanced up at me with a smug and self-satisfied look on his face as I gingerly picked up the slipper by as small a corner as I could to avoid some unknown contamination from a stranger's foot. I was about to mockingly berate Brian for losing his edge and not bringing a pair when I noticed the other one just outside the cat flap in the garden. Maybe he was just catching his breath from the effort of heaving the first one into the house.

Our newish neighbours were a lovely couple that we'd got to know as well as any neighbours do through odd pleasantries exchanged over the fence. The man of the house certainly seemed like the type who might own this type of slipper so I made an effort to look out for him later that day. I finally spotted him in the garden and put on my most apologetic face and took Brian's hard-won bounty outside with me.

'Hello, how are you?' I asked by way of warming him up.

'Fine, thanks.' The obligatory polite answer.

'Erm, I don't suppose you've recently lost a pair of slippers, have you? I'm afraid our cat, Brian, might have stolen them from your house.'

'No, I haven't, but when we got up this morning our budgie cage was tipped over on its side.' Uh-oh.

Thankfully the bird was fine but it made up my mind once and for all that I would never investigate where Brian was going on his late night foraging trips. It seemed he might be doing more than just stealing toys and footwear. But his exploits didn't end there. He teamed up with Badger for one spectacular assault, possibly to get me back for throwing his new hard-won slippers away.

The house we'd moved into was in an area of Cheltenham near to a warren of small roads of little terraced houses. Joe's surfing friend, Pete, lived a few hundred yards away through a maze of interconnecting, quiet streets. By this time we'd got into a neat routine of walking Pan and Badger round our block last thing at night before bed and the intrepid Brian loved to come too. This was all fine until we wanted to walk to Pete's house one night for a few drinks.

We didn't even think about Brian as we set off but as we heard the distinctive clatter of the cat flap we looked at each other and groaned to see Brian skipping along to catch us up. We thought he'd realise we were going somewhere new and get scared and go home, so we just ignored him and waited for him to scarper. Soon enough we got to Pete's door and there was Brian waiting patiently while we knocked.

Once inside it was obvious he was distinctly uncomfortable in his new surroundings and eventually, when I couldn't bear his uneasiness anymore, I said I'd walk the boys and him home and try to come back without him. I got to the house and opened the front door and we all trooped in. I quickly ushered the confused dogs back out of the front door, slammed it shut and legged it before Brian could get out the flap and round the house. It isn't really normal behaviour for a twenty-something to run like a headless chicken and the immediate effect was to make the dogs think this was a bloody brilliant game. They started leaping and barking and trying to nip me as I sprinted down the street. This was, at best, a bit annoying, but then Badger decided to try to have a go at it from the front. In so doing, he got in front of my legs and stopped dead, broadside to me. I'm by no means fleet of foot but going from full tilt to zero miles an hour with a thigh-high dog as the cause resulted in me being spectacularly catapulted about three metres through the air and landing like a schoolchild in the playground.

No longer being a pliable schoolchild, and not having actually fallen over for well over a decade, I crashed to the ground, with my dignity as shredded as my hands. I jumped up, cursed Badger as lividly but quietly as I could in case anyone was watching, pretended my hands didn't hurt like mad with a stinging sensation I'd not experienced since primary school, looked round to see if anyone had seen me and tried to walk off as if nothing had happened. I suppose I should have been grateful that Brian, who had started the whole sorry affair, had actually stayed put during all this and not turned up winding round my legs as I started wincingly picking the gravel out of my palms. In fact, I bet if I'd looked back at the house he would probably have been sitting with Nigel at one of the bedroom windows, watching the whole debacle and chuckling happily to himself. Bloody animals!

As well as acclimatising to the oddities of my clients, one thing I soon found I would have to get used to if I was to survive in small-animal practice was being savaged by the animals. Apart from the monumental kick in the bladder by the cow, I'd come through the smaller-animal aspects of Dulverton pretty unscathed but my very busy job in Cheltenham was about to change that. One of the saddest things about being a vet is that, although you go into the job because you absolutely adore animals and want to try to help them, they don't often see it that way. Virtually every time they visit us they are put in a room full of other odd, unknown or potentially predatory animals and then taken to another weird-smelling room where someone they hardly ever see does unspeakable things to them, usually culminating in either something up their bum or an injection. Never mind if only they could talk, I've always wished they could *understand*, so I could explain that it's all for their own good. Add to this the fact that they usually have to endure this experience when they're in pain or feeling under the weather. Or, if they're well, they were probably expecting a nice walk and the last place they wanted to end up was at our place for a vaccination. It's no wonder that sometimes they strike back and in truth it's probably all credit to the animal kingdom that they let us get away with as much as we do.

Whenever they think about vicious animals, I imagine that most people immediately conjure up an image of a huge, scary dog, but, as I've pointed out before, while these can be terrifying, they're usually the easiest to deal with. For a start you're usually prepared because of your preconceived ideas, but also big dogs are often easy to muzzle and you can use manpower to bodily restrain them and, if that doesn't work, you can use sedatives given at arm's length into a muscle as far away from the biting end as you can get. Try this with miniature dogs or rodents and you will have much more trouble. And as for cats, forget it, they've won before you even start trying. You can get muzzles for cats but the problem is that vicious cats tend to come out fighting and they have pointy weapons on what seems like every inch of their body so getting the muzzle on can be as difficult as doing whatever you wanted to do in the first place. In fact it's only their four feet and their head that are spiky but, when you take into account the agility and lightning speed of cats, the claws and teeth may as well be all over their body because wherever you try to get hold of them, at least one appendage will get you. The best veterinary nurses you can have are those who can hold evil cats. It's usually a combination of a good, firm hold and then the use of a hefty bosom to pin the cat down, putting the claws out of action while you try to get some form of sedation into the creature. Most pet cats are not like this at all of course, but if you do any charity work spaying and castrating feral cats you need great nurses. Ray was one such nurse I worked with but there were a couple of characters that got the better of our dream team despite her expertise. The first was a cat. I have a clear picture of him in my head; jet black, long-haired and pure devil! He was a stray but not properly feral, so we hadn't sedated him immediately because he'd brilliantly lulled us into a false sense of security by being quite placid on first contact. But all that niceness disappeared in a split second when we tried to restrain him for his anaesthetic injection and he turned into a spitting fireball. Ray's instincts had been honed by years of these kinds of encounters and her reflexes were themselves catlike. As soon as the first lash came from the paw the cat was immediately and very effectively bosom-pinned to the table and his head pointed in the other direction away from me. I smiled at her with heartfelt gratitude and took hold of the paw again to try to give the injection into the vein. In a feat of incredible strength and with awesome speed the cat reacted as if Ray wasn't even there and turned straight round and bit me to the full depth of his canine teeth through both sides of my hand, tendons one side and that big fleshy thumb muscle the other.

When you get badly bitten the shock is quite odd and the real pain doesn't start until later. It hurt, there was no doubt of that at the time, but the sight of the four, centimetre-deep, holes in my hand had me paralysed. Ray had the beast in a wire basket in about a fifth of a second and was mortified that I'd been got. I couldn't complain because she'd saved me from dozens of others since we'd started working together. We injected the cat through the bars with an intramuscular sedative and while we waited for him to succumb to these wonderful drugs I went off to wash my wounds and feel sorry for myself. Some hours later my whole hand was throbbing like a cartoon thumb whacked with a hammer and it had gone a very off-putting colour. All I could think about was my friend Jon, who'd been scratched by a cat on his index finger and it had become so badly infected that he'd almost lost the finger and needed surgery to flush out all his tendons. I had rather melodramatic visions of my hand falling off and asked the boss if he thought I should go to hospital. Not being the world's most sensitive man he told me to pull myself together and carry on working, and of course my hand didn't get infected, although by then I was secretly hoping it would just to prove him wrong!

Our other humdinger of an unexpected candidate came soon afterwards and was a very sweet and fluffy-looking tiny poodle. Sadly, many small dogs are born with kneecaps that slip in and out of joint through a combination of odd leg shapes and inbreeding, and there is a range of severity. Some are very painful but others hardly seem to be noticed, usually because they're the loosest ones and are just floating in the breeze. Either way, they can cause a lot of problems and often need surgery to tighten the joint, deepen the groove the kneecap should sit in or even realign the bones in the leg to reduce the wear and tear that leads to arthritis when joints aren't doing what they're supposed to.

We'd admitted this tiny scrap of a dog for X-rays but we did have an inkling he might be more trouble than his diminutive size suggested: his owner had warned us that she hadn't managed to get him clipped yet because he was too aggressive to be done. As any poodle owner will tell you, the breed sheds hardly any hair at all so they need clipping to keep their gorgeous locks under control. As a result of having never been trimmed, this tiny ball of fur looked like the kind of bobble that kids make to go on their hats. Being black to boot, the dog seemed to have no definition to any part of his body, and his face was completely masked by his amazing Rastafarian fringe.

The dog seemed pretty happy in his kennel after he'd been admitted and we wondered if his owner had been sucked in by the manipulative young thing until we tried to get him out. I was chatting absent-mindedly to Ray as I reached in to lift him out and without a single bit of a warning he turned into a mini Tasmanian devil and leapt for my hand, snarling and growling like fury. My also-well-honed reflexes whipped my hands away before he got me and I snapped the cage door shut and leaned against the opposite wall of the small kennel room. We both heaved a sigh of relief and laughed nervously as we looked at the now quiet little mouse in his kennel. But we had a problem. The dog was so small and so incredibly savage, and it was so difficult to make out one part of his body from another, that I wasn't sure how we were actually going to get him out. I had no choice but to go and get the gauntlets. These are a must in any practice. Great for exotics and birds of prey, these large, long, and very thick leather gloves are also a finger saver from many a cat and dog attack. I approached the cage with more than a little trepidation and Ray was standing by with a small cat basket for me to 'pop' the dog into once I'd got hold of him. As I opened the door and tried to block the space like an ice hockey goalie he flew into a rage and simply started spinning every which way, furiously gnashing his teeth.

In his wild mop of hair all you could see was a ball of fur and blurred flashes of pure white as his little choppers sought to sink in to anything they could find. If I hadn't been so scared I might have seen the funny side of the spectacle.

I had to just go for it in the end, so I shut my eyes, made a lunge into the depths and scooped the flying furball out into the basket. Ray snapped the lid shut and we both burst out laughing at our being almost bested by this dog, which was actually about the same size as a large guinea pig! With some chemical help the rest of the investigation was a lot more relaxed for everyone concerned, including our patient, and I knew we were going to have to have words with his owner if he was going to come in for orthopaedic surgery and multiple post-op appointments. Either he needed serious behavioural help or I needed to hand my notice in or make sure it wasn't me on duty next time he came in!

The fact is that his owner knew what he was like and had given us fair warning. When I told her about our adventures with him that day she was mortally embarrassed. Most people are the same and are very reasonable, as you might expect, when they own an animal that is likely to savage you as soon as look at you. Most are a little abashed at the behaviour, to say the least, and will help you however they can. But not all.

Whenever I have anything but the smallest of dogs in I try to avoid putting them on the table. I think most dogs find the table a very odd place to be: they are much more comfortable and less stressed on the floor. This makes for happy dogs but it also means I spend a lot of my time crawling around on the floor and talking to people from my knees like an anxious lover about to propose. Whenever I have an animal in my care I always want to do a full examination if possible, to make sure I don't miss anything the owner might not have noticed.

One patient I saw was a beautiful liver-and-white pointer with a very docile face and a very relaxed owner. She was only in for a vaccination and I was chatting to him and stroking her ears as I did so. I finished what we were saying and got down on my knees in front of this calmly sitting dog. I looked at her eyes and ears and felt all round her face to check her lymph nodes were normal, felt down her chest and then picked up the end of my stethoscope and put the ear pieces in. I leaned forward and slid the stethoscope onto the side of her chest to start checking her heart. It was at this point that with not a growl or snarl of warning she sprang at my face, teeth bared, and snapped. My face, at the time, was about six inches from her nose and it was a very close call. My cat-like reflexes had made me retreat before I even consciously registered what had happened. To my absolute amazement her owner didn't bat an eyelid as he said, 'Sorry. She does that.'

I finished my exam from a healthier, safer, standing distance and vaccinated her without further injury but it was one of those infuriating situations where afterwards you think of all the things you should have said. I'd been so shocked at the time I didn't say anything. I just smiled fixedly like I had a bad case of lockjaw and carried on with the job. It was only later that I contemplated how close I'd been to being badly bitten in the face and he *knew* she was likely to do it. I was telling a friend about it later and she suggested I should have unexpectedly lashed out and slapped him hard in the face and then said, 'Oh sorry. I do that.' I laughed a lot at the image and the feeling of sweet revenge but I didn't think it would be a very good way to keep client relations up and had a feeling that the Royal College might not see it too favourably either.

Despite these little altercations, which are after all to be expected in my line of work, I was loving the change from farm animals to purely pets, not least because I could be a girly wuss and stay indoors in the cold weather. It was also soon after moving that I got one of the most amazing letters I've ever received. *Vets In Practice* was turning out not just to be popular in Britain but had 'gone global'. This sounds very grand and I might be overstating it but there's no doubt that the show became enormously loved in Northern Europe. One day at work I received a little parcel from a couple called Bart and Valerie in Belgium. Apparently it is tradition in Belgium to send out little presents when you have a baby and they had sent me a little gift along with a beautiful photo of their daughter. Why? Because they had named her after me. To this day this is still one of the most touching and flattering things I've ever experienced. I felt totally humbled and overwhelmed. I wrote back to express my shock and gratitude and wish them all the best. Quite recently I tried to get back in touch, curious as to how my little namesake was doing, but my letter was returned because they had moved. So if you're called Emma, you're Belgian and your mum and dad named you after a silly old vet on the TV, I'd love to hear from you!

One of our most colourful clients during my time at that surgery in Cheltenham was a man called Dave. He was probably in his mid-twenties and, without meaning to sound *too* unkind, he had a certain aroma, which always accompanied him into the surgery. Vets are pretty immune to most smells and bodily functions, but the aroma of ingrained damp and dirt can outdo even the most evil of animal smells. All vets' surgeries are armed with little bottles of odour-neutralising sprays for events like anal gland emptying but every time we knew Dave was coming in we would have one behind the reception desk to be liberally sprayed round after his departure.

Dave was the very proud owner of a pedigree chow called Duke. For those of you who don't know, these are very striking dogs in that they are about the size of a small and slim Labrador but look three times the size they actually are because they have incredibly thick, dense and long fur. In Duke's case, this coat trapped the odour of Dave and his house very effectively indeed.

I suspect they are lovely pets but in the surgery nearly all the chows I've come across have a very strong propensity to yap incessantly like overgrown lapdogs the whole time they are in. When you are trying to examine them or have a serious discussion with their owner, this can make life a little difficult, to say the least. This particular chow was a world-class yapper and also an uncastrated male. Try as I might, even my powers of getting testicles off most things that come through the door had so far failed to persuade Dave to remove his boy's crown jewels. This meant that a visit from the duo went something like this: the surgery had very large front windows so afforded a good view a long way down the street. Dave would be spotted approaching the surgery with Duke, who would be skipping lightly along at his side. We would subconsciously hold our breath as they entered the surgery to try to delay the onslaught on our olfactory nerves for as long as possible. Duke would immediately and without fail start yapping in a startlingly high-pitched tone and start urinating up every corner of every piece of furniture in the surgery and I would promise myself once again that I would get the nuts off this dog if was my last act of veterinary surgery. The constant territory-marking combined with the ridiculously impractical coat meant that the whole of Duke's undercarriage was a mass of yellow, urine-soaked, matted fur. Visits from this pair were not usually a savoury highlight of the working day so you can imagine our horror at the realisation one day that there was a very strong likelihood that Duke was properly poorly and needed admitting for tests and possible surgery.

Duke had started vomiting and it had carried on for a day or two with him managing to keep nothing down, all the while trying to eat but bringing up totally undigested food. He was pretty bright in himself but was starting to lose the skip in his stride and Dave was really worried. These signs, combined with his young age, made an intestinal foreign body quite high up on our list of possible causes. As many a dog owner will know, dogs are happy to eat an incredible array of items that range from the very unappetising, like poo (they don't seem to mind if it's their own or anyone else's), to the quite impossible to imagine, in the case of a famous dog within the veterinary world which managed to swallow a six-inch, wooden-handled carving knife and not show many signs of trouble for some weeks afterwards.

We admitted Duke, ran some blood tests to make sure nothing untoward was going on from a medical point of view, and started him on a drip because he was getting dangerously dehydrated as he could keep nothing down. The bloods showed a high white cell count and not much else, which could have been a sign of a simple upset stomach but in this case made our suspicion of a foreign body more likely. My next job was to anaesthetise him so I could have a good feel of his abdomen and take some X-rays. Finding foreign bodies in intestines can be notoriously and surprisingly difficult without 'going in'. Many things that dogs eat have an organic composition like peach stones, socks, rubber balls and such like, so they can appear exactly the same colour as the soft tissues of the abdomen or like the intestines themselves on an X-ray. Only inorganic things like metal and mineral-rich rocks give you the classic, cracking foreign-body films every vet wants to see. You can look for telltale signs, though, even if the object itself is hiding, so X-rays are always needed to rule out other problems and also to see if you've got a corker of a find to add to the veterinary hall of fame!

Snaffled oddities can sit quite happily in the stomach for very long periods of time but the real danger comes when they try to pass through the small intestine. The name gives it away – it's small. The stomach can stretch to a large size and accommodate many things but with normal food, after some digestion, the next phase is to be squeezed into the small bowel, which is about an inch wide on average. It has some give, of course, but nothing compared to what some dogs expect to get through there. As the offending object passes into this narrow passageway it gets stuck sooner or later and gradually becomes inextricably wedged. The normal pulsing waves of the gut which move food from your mouth all the way through to your bottom simply serve to wedge it in further and further. The small intestine stretches way too much when this happens, and the blood supply gets cut off, which can lead to rapid and catastrophic breakdown of the gut wall, peritonitis and death. It's certainly not something to be taken lightly.

As always, right at the start, we'd asked Dave if there was anything he thought Duke might have eaten or if anything odd had gone missing from the house. The most diligent owners in the world can't watch their dog 24–7 and it's rare in these cases that you get a positive answer and Dave was no exception. I tried not to imagine what his house was like, or how much would have to go missing before he noticed it, and tried to get on with the job in hand. As is often the case, once Duke was anaesthetised and the muscles of his abdomen were totally relaxed I could quite easily feel a definite lump. As it turned out we could also see the thing on our X-rays, because of its shape more than its make-up. It seemed to be u-shaped, like a cross section of a small paper cup, and was wedged firmly in his small intestine, not far from the outlet of the stomach. The reason these animals stay so bright and keep eating for a while is because the obstruction hasn't caused any damage yet, but food has nowhere to go so it has to come back up the way it went down, largely unchanged.

His only option was emergency surgery to get the thing, whatever it was, out, before the gut got further damaged and might need sections removing. These ops are just the sort of thing I absolutely love. They undeniably need doing, they are life-saving and they also require very small and intricate stitching of soft tissues, which is what I like best. They also have the added bonus that you get to try to guess what's in there and at the end of it, if all goes well, you get a great souvenir to give the owner to remember it by.

Luckily for me, apart from his personal hygiene, Dave was a great owner and had picked up on Duke's problem quickly before too much damage was done, so the surgery was as straightforward as these ops ever are. The object was very obvious when we got him opened up and a simple incision over the top of it had it popped out in no time at all. I stitched the hole in the gut, squeezed very gently to check for leaks, which you definitely don't want, and then checked the whole and considerable length of the rest of the gut to be sure there wasn't anything else lurking that we hadn't spotted. Once I was satisfied there would be no further surprises I stitched up the muscles and skin so that Duke could start his recovery and we could examine our bounty.

We still weren't really sure what it was after it had been washed and dried. It looked just like it did on X-ray but we could see now that it was made of black rubber and did indeed look like a small cup with no handle. When Dave came to see Duke later that day he knew immediately what it was and apparently we had solved an ongoing family mystery of some days – the odd and sudden disappearance of the end of his granddad's walking stick. A very satisfying day all round but there was something else about it that had me smiling.

Although I hadn't managed to 'slip' with my scalpel and 'accidentally' remove Duke's testicles, I had had to shave and clean the entirety of his undercarriage for the surgery, so for a few weeks at least he might be free of the clagging smell of his own urine, even if we couldn't rid him of the smell of his sweet-natured owner.

Interesting cases like Duke's and brilliant characters like Dave were abundant when I moved to Cheltenham. I'd found a job with a decent salary and a good rota, I loved my patients and the nurses too and we had some absolutely wonderful clients. I also knew that small-animal practice was definitely right for me. But as time went by I found myself becoming more and more unhappy. I wish I could regale you at length about all the fun and interesting times I had but the truth is that I've largely blanked a lot of it out because I became so desperately low during the eighteen months I worked there. Now, when I look back, I sometimes can't believe I stayed as long as I did.

There was nothing I could really put my finger on, which is probably why it was such a slow and gradual drop in my morale, but it started to become more and more clear that Barry and I were simply not destined to get on. This might sound a silly reason to leave a good job where I got on well with everyone else, but anyone who's had a 'personality clash' with someone will understand, I'm sure. The fact is that no money in the world could compensate for the dread I was starting to feel at going to work, and as the months went by I came to realise that for the sake of my sanity I would have to leave. Joe and I had talked about me leaving the job before but I'd tried to stay on there; we both had student debts to pay off, Joe was working part-time and we had just bought our house, so we simply couldn't afford for me to leave. Eventually, though, we both came to realise that I was heading for a nervous breakdown if I stayed, so on one very happy day I finally handed in my notice and felt as if the weight of the world had been lifted from my shoulders. It was time to move on again.

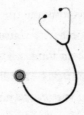

Chapter 7

Stick it to me

I needed to find a job pretty quickly or we'd be out on our ears, and I couldn't work in the immediate vicinity because, like many vets' contracts, mine had a clause in it which prevented this to stop me potentially poaching clients. I heard through Joe's boss that a small practice just up the motorway in Tewkesbury was a one-man band who was desperate for some time off and therefore needed some part-time help. We did our sums and it would mean that we would lose about £14,000 a year from our combined income, but I felt my sanity and happiness were well worth it so I made some enquiries.

I made an appointment to have a look around the place and chat to Simon, the boss, and of course the BBC came with me. The practice had quite an odd layout, having been shoehorned into a small house, but it had a lovely intimate feel and I knew I'd get good continuity with clients even being part-time because there would only be the two of us. Working three days a week and some Saturday mornings meant that I would almost always be able to ask people to come back on my days for follow-ups. To be honest, no matter what the place was like, I was out of options and when Simon said he was happy to have me I was over the moon and suddenly found myself looking forward to getting started. My smile returned and the clouds of the last few months seemed to clear.

I always felt a little self-conscious being followed around by a film crew whenever I first went somewhere. I never wanted to appear like a prima donna and I knew that some people would assume that was what I was like before getting to know the real and hopefully very down-to-earth me. It seemed that a very scary nurse in my new job was going to be one of those. Her name was Julie and when I first started work there I was terrified of her, mostly because of her incredible sneer. She had this way of looking at me that made me feel like I should prostrate myself before her and ask for forgiveness even though I hadn't done anything wrong. She was brilliant at her job, a devoted animal lover and, at about five foot nothing, nonetheless seemed to be ten foot tall in her domination of the practice and everyone who worked there, Simon and me included. She was also wonderful with clients – as long as they were animal lovers too – and Lord help those who weren't.

At the vet's we often get clients in as a couple but sometimes you feel that one of them has been dragged along, possibly against their free will, and it's usually the husband. Some will get forced into the consultation too but some are simply fulfilling taxi duties, or are there to pay the bill, and are left to amuse themselves in the waiting room while the wife talks serious health matters with the vet without fear of interruption by the second-class citizen of the household. One such unfortunate man was left in the waiting room, with the diminutive Julie sitting behind the reception desk, no doubt looking harmless enough. The man did what most people do in those circumstances and started glancing at the numerous posters on the walls and probably started feeling like the uncomfortable silence in such a small, enclosed space needed breaking with some small talk. He spotted a poster about fly strike in rabbits.

Fly strike is an absolutely horrible condition of rabbits that we see every summer without fail unfortunately. Many rabbits are kept in less than ideal conditions as children's pets and tend to get stuck in a hutch at the end of the garden and largely forgotten about. In the summer, if the rabbit is in dirty conditions or has poo round its bottom, then flies get attracted, lay their eggs and the poor rabbits get literally eaten alive by maggots. They're some of the worst things we consistently see at the surgery and it is totally preventable if only people would look after their animals well and check them every single day and twice a day through the summer. The shocking headline of the poster was designed to catch the eye and read 'FLY STRIKE KILLS RABBITS!' The man obviously thought he'd struck chit-chat gold with this and turned to Julie and said, 'That fly strike stuff. Do you sell that here? I've got terrible trouble with wild rabbits eating the garden and I'd love to kill them.' There was a short, stony silence and, I imagine, an Olympic champion of a sneer before he was verbally battered to the size of a walnut on exactly what fly strike was, what a horrible death it caused, how he shouldn't kill anything living at all and if he did want to then shouting about it at a vet's surgery of all places wasn't the way to make friends and influence people.

I'm sure by the time his wife finally emerged from my consulting room he was practically climbing the walls to get away from the ice queen and as they left I got the full story from Julie. How was he to know that she had about ten rescue rabbits at the time and their whole garden was devoted to them? Poor bugger. By this time I'd well and truly got used to Julie's ways and loved her wicked sense of humour and she had decided that I wasn't all that bad too so we had a very good chuckle amongst ourselves at the start of what was to become a brilliant and enduring friendship.

Folly Gardens, as the practice was called, turned out to be a great move for me. I've always loved working in a small surgery environment because you get a great combination of independence and client continuity but there's usually good support in the background if you need it. I think for young graduates they can be challenging environments to work in but in the long run they can make you stronger vets because you can't always fall back on someone else whenever you encounter a problem. The people you work with in small places also make a huge difference and in Julie I had found a soulmate who shared my passion for the job, had the professionalism needed to be mature when things were serious but who could be guaranteed to share my facile sense of humour and make me smile when the stresses and strains of the job all got a bit too much.

We shared a lot of experiences and one of the most memorable happened pretty soon after I started at Folly Gardens and tested the nurses and me to some new and unexplored limits. Elwood was a giant of a cat. I've always been a huge fan of the film *The Blues Brothers* so I immediately warmed to his owner when I recognised that he and his brother were named after Jake and Elwood Blues. Elwood was as beautiful as he was big. He was jet black and had a coat as sleek as a panther's. He stalked onto the table out of his basket, calmly settled onto his haunches like the Sphinx and immediately dominated the room. He seemed to be in for a fairly innocuous reason. His 'mum' reported that he'd lost his voice and he was normally a very vocal cat. Cats can get sore throats for a number of reasons, just like humans, and my first thought was that he had some kind of infection. But, as always, a top to toe examination was the way forward and this revealed something straight away that the owner had not noticed. All his claws were scuffed and ragged. Because cats retract their claws many owners never see them, so it wasn't odd that she hadn't noticed them and, to be honest, she was being incredibly astute bringing him in for something like a voice change.

Scuffed claws are very often a classic sign in cats of a road accident. It has always amazed me how many cats get hit by cars and survive, often relatively unscathed. Of course not all are so lucky and certain injuries are very common, like broken pelvises, damaged tails and broken jaws, depending on where the impact has occurred. But virtually all of them have scuffed claws, because they get dragged and instinctively the claws come out to grip the road and oppose the motion of the car. I was very suspicious after I'd seen his claws and felt carefully over his whole skeleton. He had no outward signs of any other injuries at all. No fractures, no cuts, no bruises and he didn't seem to be in any discomfort. He just sat on the table like the calmest customer in the world and let me do whatever I liked. When I listened to his chest more clues began to emerge. I could hear his heart but it was very muffled and his breathing was shallower and a bit faster than I would have expected for such a calm and huge feline.

We needed to X-ray him to be sure of what was going on and I printed out the consent form for his owner to sign. Elwood didn't object in the slightest when we carried him gently through to the kennels and placed him in a cage. He took it all in his stride and just relaxed on his bed, surveying his surroundings. After morning surgery had finished we set up the X-ray machine and got him out. He was fast becoming our favourite patient ever because he was just so good and practically proffered his paw for the anaesthetic injection.

We took X-rays of both his chest and his abdomen to be sure, but his problem was clear from the first one. He had a ruptured diaphragm. The diaphragm is a muscular sheet that separates the contents of the chest from the abdomen. It is a dome shape at rest and when it flattens out it makes a vacuum in the chest, expands the lungs and draws breath in. As it relaxes, the chest collapses back to a small size and the air is squeezed back out. All this your body takes care of so you never have to give it a second thought until it goes wrong. What wonderful machines we are.

The chest is pretty elastic and has a fair amount of give in it, so when a huge impact happens, like being hit square in the chest by a car, the ribcage will flex as much as possible but the force has to be transmitted somewhere. Some of the time the ribs will break but in some cases, like Elwood's, the force gets dissipated into the abdomen by the diaphragm rupturing open. The X-rays showed that a large portion of his liver and a lot of his small intestines and stomach had moved up through the tear into his chest cavity, and his lungs were compressed to a fraction of their normal size. It was astounding that he was outwardly as well as he was.

I felt an odd mixture of excitement and fear. I love soft tissue surgery but I'd never had to operate on one of these before. In order to repair the diaphragm I would have to go into his chest to his heart and lungs and pull all his organs back into place. I'd have to carefully stitch the tear in the diaphragm and try to restore an airtight seal. I'd have to put a chest drain in, which I'd also never done before, so that we could gradually remove all the air that would result from the surgery, and so that his lungs would reinflate gradually and not get damaged. As soon as I opened him up and allowed air in, his lungs would collapse because the vacuum would be broken and we would have to breathe for him using our anaesthetic circuit. Julie was a fully qualified nurse and was trained in positive pressure ventilation, as it's called, but had never actually done it. This left Sarah, our lovely trainee, to scrub up and help me hold the organs out of the way while I repaired the diaphragm. Something she'd never done before either. Gulp. And of course the BBC crew was there to film the whole thing. Big gulp.

I phoned Elwood's owner and told her what needed to be done and told her that the surgery was certainly not without its risks. It had to be done, though, because of the enormous internal damage, and she gave consent for us to get straight on with it while he was still anaesthetised. We got everything we needed assembled as quickly as possible because time was of the essence, as ever in surgery, and we got started. With Elwood on his back, body clipped and scrubbed from neck to pelvis, I cut down through the skin and layers of thin tissue to get to what we call the white line. This is where the muscles of the two halves of the body meet and would be the middle of a six-pack if you were lucky enough to have a boyfriend who hadn't lost his to beer years before you met him. The white line is a fibrous kind of join with hardly any blood supply, so it's perfect as a place to get into the abdomen, with little bleeding and good strong tissue to stitch back together.

We knew that, as soon as I went through the white line, air would rush in and collapse his lungs, so I told Julie to get ready to take over his breathing. There was a sucking sound as my scalpel popped through and Julie immediately started using the bag of the anaesthetic circuit to slowly and rhythmically pump air into his lungs. It was now that I could see with my own eyes the level of the internal damage. There was a huge tear in the diaphragm and I started very gently pulling his abdominal organs back into the right body cavity. As the guts, then the stomach and finally the liver came back, I was left with a view straight into his open chest and I looked on in slight disbelief at his heart, which was beating away as if nothing at all was wrong. I could see his lungs expanding and contracting with each of Julie's breaths. It was one of the most incredible moments of my career. I reached in to pull the last bit of tissue through and my fingertips touched his heart, which pulsed against me. It was amazing.

As quickly and carefully as I could I started the big job of closing the hole in his diaphragm. It was painstaking and intricate work but was everything about soft-tissue surgery that I love. Finally I had everything back where it should be, the diaphragm was intact again and it was time to stop the breaths and see if Elwood's body would resume that most important of jobs for itself. I made sure everything was as it should be from my end and then Sarah and I pulled our hands out and I told Julie to stop the compressions. I can tell you now that the three of us and the whole film crew held our breath. After a few long seconds, as Elwood suddenly and wonderfully took a great big breath on his own, we all breathed an enormous unified sigh of relief. It didn't take long to stitch up his abdomen and put his chest drain in and then it was up to him and Father Time. I stayed at the surgery into the early hours of the following morning to periodically draw air out of his chest through the drain to allow his lungs to gradually reinflate and, when there seemed to be virtually nothing coming out, I said goodnight to him and made my weary way home.

The next morning I drove to work about four hours after I'd left but the adrenalin was pumping and there wasn't a hint of tiredness about me. I opened the surgery door with more than a little trepidation and part of me was dreading the convoluted, short walk from the front door to the kennel room to see how Elwood was. Or wasn't. As it turned out, I didn't need to walk through the surgery to get my answer. As soon as I pushed open the front door I could hear a loud, incredible, wonderful, booming meow and a huge smile spread across my face. When I got to his kennel Elwood was climbing up the bars trying to bat his notes off the door of the cage and was quite clearly saying he was feeling very well indeed. I opened the door and gave him a huge fuss and a cuddle, which he deigned to accept, purring like a tractor and winding back and forth in front of me. I offered him a small bowl of special food because I needed to know if he'd be willing to eat and because I couldn't let him go home until I knew his intestines were working and happy. I didn't need to worry because he practically inhaled the food before I could even put the bowl down and carried on winding round me purring and meowing. Later that day he had his drain removed and went home with a very happy owner and leaving behind a *very* happy vet.

As it turned out, Elwood wasn't going to be my only foray into an animal's chest while I worked at Folly Gardens. Soon afterwards I met a dog called Twiggy, a lovely, skinny, leggy and slightly shaggy lurcher who'd been named after the model. (They apparently shared a lot of the same attributes, although the human Twiggy might not appreciate the 'slightly shaggy' comment. In this same vein I also know a Great Dane who had such a lovely flat and smooth tummy as a youngster that her male owner just had to name her Britney, as in Spears.) Twiggy was rushed in one day when the BBC were twiddling their thumbs and suddenly they had something to get excited about. She had been playing in the park and had become impaled on a stick.

Before I go on I must digress for a few moments. If there is one thing I'd like you to take away from reading this book it is this: DO NOT THROW STICKS FOR YOUR DOG. This is probably a big surprise to many of you because it is the epitome of a lovely walk in the woods, but sticks kill and seriously injure numerous dogs every year. The stick gets thrown, bounces, goes end over end and your dog, at full pelt, runs straight onto the end of it, mouth open, as it tumbles on the ground. There are many ways the stick can go but most of them end up lodged in the mouth or throat somewhere and they can go straight through the back of the pharynx and up into the brain in the worst cases.

As I tuck my soapbox quietly under my arm again, I'll get back to the story of Twiggy. Now her owners knew about the dangers of these harmless-looking things and had a strict policy of not throwing them, but Twiggy had other ideas and was practically inseparable from sticks. Having given up trying to get her owners to oblige, she had decided to just play with a stick by herself. She'd spied a good-looking one in the distance and had torn off in hot pursuit and at full lurcher speed, which is pretty awesome to watch if ever you get the chance, and pretty scary if they do it straight towards you in the park!

As she neared the holy grail of stickdom she slammed the brakes on and leapt on to it but in her haste she ended up standing on one end of it, bouncing the stick upwards. The momentum carried her chest straight onto the other end of it. She'd screamed and the stick broke off and fell away as she tried to run off. She hobbled in agony back to her owners. They'd seen what had happened and she had a horrible hole in her side, so they'd just headed straight for us as quickly as they could.

When they arrived, Twiggy and her owners all looked in shock and she was in a lot of pain, which worsened when I went anywhere near the wounded area. I certainly needed to admit her and we took her in straight away and sent her owners home for a strong coffee or maybe a brandy. We gave Twiggy something for the pain and got her started on antibiotics because of the risk of infection from the penetration of the stick. I hooked her up to a drip and we anaesthetised her so that I could explore the wound and find out the extent of the injuries.

The hole in her chest wall was full of splinters and bits of wood and I started carefully removing as much debris as I could possibly find. I probed into the hole with a sterile instrument to see which direction the tract went in. What often happens with chest injuries like this is that the object breaks the skin and then travels under the skin until it hits a rib, which then deflects it into the chest itself. In Twiggy's case the stick had gone along about two rib spaces and then did a sudden right-angled turn into her chest. I had to go all the way in, to be sure that everything had been removed and right inside I found a piece of wood about an inch long where the stick had broken off. Where Twiggy had actually been quite lucky was that the stick had taken this odd path into her chest and not gone straight through. It had actually made itself a self-sealing passage in by going under the skin first so it hadn't actually collapsed her lungs, which probably helped her survive long enough to get to us. Of course, by the nature of what I had to do, I had let some air in and I also needed to flush everything out thoroughly with saline to reduce contamination of the wound to a minimum, so Twiggy also needed a chest drain, just as Elwood had.

I sent her home later that day with her drain in place, tucked into some lovely bandages we had that had 'ouch' written all over them in different languages, which we and the owners generally loved. Her whole chest was bandaged round to cover her wounds and keep her chest drain in place and she somehow seemed diminished in size as she went away hunched and feeling very sorry for herself. Her owners had all the antibiotics and painkillers she needed and had instructions to keep on intermittently drawing air off her drain. By the time I saw her the next day she was looking pretty brilliant, all things considered, and it seemed she had had a very lucky escape. The big bonus for me, with the BBC being involved, was that I got to see the footage they shot just a week or so later when she was back in the park and once again defying gravity in that way that only whippets and lurchers seem able to do. As vets this is something we are hardly ever privy to and it was wonderful to watch her stretching out and sprinting about without a care in the world so soon after she had come to us with possibly life-threatening injuries. Of course the BBC were doubly happy because they hadn't missed the irony of the fact that a dog called Twiggy had been impaled on a stick.

The film crew did love the quirky, tabloid-style names they came up with for the stories they planned to show and 'grilled pheasant' was another one that got their creative spark going that summer. When I worked in Dulverton I was in a huge hunting and shooting area and the pheasant population was enormous, but in all my time there I don't think I ever got brought an injured pheasant to treat. Maybe it was the kind of place that injured game birds get their necks swiftly wrung and either go in the pot or get tossed in a hedgerow. However, the majority of the public, who aren't familiar with such practicalities, are mortified when they hit something with their car and many go to extraordinary lengths to try to find help, whatever the poor creature happens to be. Sadly, what often happens is that shock and adrenalin can make even a very badly injured animal run away, never to be seen again while it slopes off to die somewhere and the poor driver never knows quite where it went. In the case of 'grilled pheasant', the driver had the exact opposite of this problem.

It was a beautiful sunny day and we were having an unusually quiet and relaxing afternoon. The film crew had a pile of trashy magazines to read and I was catching up on notes and phone calls and lab results when a very distressed-looking young man came barging through the front door. He breathlessly asked for help and gestured that we needed to follow him to the car park. The crew grabbed all their gear and as we trooped out the man told me that he'd hit a pheasant about three miles away from the surgery, and I was just wondering why he couldn't bring it in to the surgery as he'd obviously stopped to pick it up, when he explained that it was wedged into the front grill of his car and he couldn't get it out. He was pretty sure it was still alive so he'd driven really slowly for three miles until he found the nearest vet.

I'd been taught many things at vet school but bird-car extraction was not one of them. I crouched down and peered slightly disbelievingly into the front of the car and, sure enough, wedged between the grill and the radiator, was a slightly dazed and confused-looking but most definitely alive pheasant, blinking slowly in the shadows. The whole bird had been sucked bodily into the space between the bars and seemed to have somehow not had a wing out of place to be damaged by the impact. I didn't have a clue about how to get the bird out, but the logical part of my brain told me that it had got in there through the gap so therefore it must come out. So I just pulled harder than the man had and out it came. The man looked very relieved indeed and I told him we'd see what we could do and thanked him for the extraordinary lengths he'd gone to to bring the bird in. In hindsight he didn't really have a choice about taking the bird with him but, even so, he'd been very sweet about the whole thing.

Wildlife doesn't appreciate handling or being in captivity and, as a rule, if you can pick a wild animal up without it escaping then there is a fifty–fifty chance that it is not going to pull through, no matter what you do. The pheasant was very weak, shocked and could barely even lift its head. I didn't hold out much hope but there were no injuries I could see at all, wings and legs intact, so I had to try. We gave the bird fluids, medication for shock and antibiotics as a cover-all-your-bases tactic and put food and water in its cage. We covered the cage to make it as dark and quiet as possible, in order to reduce the stress of being surrounded by very odd people and animals as much as we could, and waited.

The next day the bird was miraculously recovered, head erect and proud and looking for all the world like he'd very much like to go now, please. As soon as I got a break in the day we all drove off into the neighbouring countryside and the crew filmed the magnificent release of the grilled pheasant. I let him out and he took off across the fields, doing that ridiculous run that pheasants do that always leaves you wondering why they don't just fly. Maybe it's because when they do take to the air so many of them get summarily shot to provide humans with an outlet for their Neanderthal cravings to pit themselves against animals! Anyway, no matter what destiny had in store for him, I'd done my bit and I felt rather pleased about the whole affair and so did the BBC.

Of course, not everyone wants to be filmed and not all stories which seem to be good television material come to an exciting climax, but the BBC thought they were onto a certain winner when Joe found a horrible-looking tumour on the ear of my beloved Badger one day.

By this time Joe had moved to a job in Carterton, near Oxford, which was an easy commute from our home in Cheltenham, and we shared the days of who had the boys at work depending on who was most likely to get time to walk them during their day. This particular night we were planning to go to my parents' house in Kent for the weekend so we'd decided that Joe would take the boys to work and then I'd drive to Carterton. We'd leave a car there and go on to Kent together. Joe had the BBC with him so I was having a very peaceful and easy day until I got the awful phone call that afternoon. As a vet it is horrible to operate on your own animals and very easy to lose your clinical judgement when they are ill. Mixed with this, I've always felt duty-bound to perform their treatments and surgeries myself because I'd simply never forgive myself if something went wrong and I hadn't. Several months previously I'd had to remove a small tumour from the edge of Badger's ear and I'd felt dreadfully sorry for him as he woozily came round wondering what had happened. The tumour itself was a thing called a histiocytoma, which is a pretty common skin tumour in young dogs and nothing to worry about. Some of these tumours get better on their own and others need removing. I'd opted to remove Badger's because as it grew it would become trickier to remove and because he was scratching at it all the time, making it bleed. I'd hated doing the surgery on 'my baby' but it had healed beautifully and all that was left was a small and unique nick in his ear where the offending lump had once been. And now Joe had found another one.

Unbeknown to me, the BBC had rigged the phone up his end to record him breaking the news to me. He told me he couldn't believe we hadn't seen it before because it was two or three times the size of the last one and was an angry red colour and really very obvious. I was devastated, firstly because my heart sank that I'd have to knock him out again, but also because I felt so guilty that I hadn't noticed it myself. Badger was often with me twenty-four hours a day and I pride myself on my keen observational skills. I got through the rest of the day in a bit of a low state and headed off to go and meet up with Joe that evening.

As soon as I arrived at the meeting place I jumped out of the car as Joe was grabbing what he needed for the weekend and the boys' stuff to transfer between cars. As he opened the boot the boys leapt out to greet me and I immediately seized upon poor Badger to inspect him. Joe had his head buried deep in the boot gathering belongings as he told me once again how aggressive-looking the mass was and how he couldn't believe we hadn't seen it before. By this time I had found the mass he was referring to, had identified it as most likely a very artificially-coloured boiled sweet which was clinging rather precariously to the fur on the edge of Badger's ear, and had plucked it off in about one second flat.

'You didn't mean this, did you?' I said as I held out the small scrap of confectionery in the palm of my hand. 'I think it's a piece of a sweet.' He stopped what he was doing, dropped the bags on the ground and inspected it. The colour drained from his face and he turned ashen. He grabbed Badger's ear and desperately searched it, and then the other one, for the awful tumour he was so sure must still be there.

'Oh my God,' he groaned, 'I even got my boss to look at it and he said it looked a bit like a sweet and it took me ages to convince him it was a tumour.'

The monumental nature of his mistake was dawning on him and he knew the BBC wanted to film the operation and my reaction and all the emotion that went with it, but mostly I suspect he knew what I was thinking.

'Please don't tell anyone,' he pleaded, 'oh no, please don't tell your dad.' My dad is a bit of a mickey-taker, to say the least, and he knew Dad would get a lot of mileage out of this one. As he raised his gaze to meet mine he knew he was scuppered because I had the biggest, happiest and most malevolent smile on my face you can imagine. My eyes twinkled with delight as I collapsed in hysterical laughter. His shoulders slumped and we climbed into the car for one of the longest journeys of his life and one of the most enjoyable of mine. All the way to Kent I would periodically burst into uncontrollable, side-splitting laughter and then try to contain myself as Joe sat and looked dejectedly out of the window.

We arrived at my mum and dad's house a couple of hours later and I think I lasted about thirty seconds before I blurted out the whole glorious story. I'd like to sound noble and genuine and say I was only happy because I was relieved Badger was OK, and not because I was revelling in someone else's misfortune, but I cannot tell a lie. It was just magic. And Dad thought so too. The BBC never did get to film the end of the story and Joe made sure they knew that, without having filmed what had happened in the car park, it *really* wasn't worth them pursuing it at all, but I'm sure they wished they could have done.

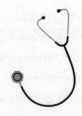

Chapter 8

Till Death Us Do Part

The television success of *Vets in Practice* and all such animal-related media relies on the human characters as well as the animals, be they unwittingly silly vets or owners in all their glorious guises. One such character that I met when I worked at Folly Gardens became a great friend and was a truly inspirational woman. Edwina had always had a love of pugs and when I knew her she had one with the very grand and literary name of Chaucer (he was the successor to the equally grandly named Gatsby). Edwina had led one of the most varied and colourful lives I've ever encountered but the first few times I met her I saw her simply as a very dignified and *very* well-spoken older lady. Being from Kent I have a bit of a commoner's accent, so compared to me Edwina spoke the Queen's English. Until I really got to know her I always felt I should be on my best behaviour and try not to drop my 't's as best I could.

After several visits to the consultation room we started to gel and I realised I needn't have been worried. Poor Chaucer was getting older and he was a bit disadvantaged because he was a rescue dog and had had an accident before Edwina took him on. The accident had left him with a permanent head tilt and only one eye, but he coped extremely well and was a stalwart character, as most pugs are. I'd really started to warm to the pair and looked forward to seeing them whenever I saw their names on the day list. I was starting to realise that each visit would not only be an encounter with a lovely client and a well-natured pet, but that there would also nearly always be a fascinating instalment from Edwina's life story in store. These were too numerous to recount here but one of my favourites was from her childhood. At about the age of ten she had been walking happily down a street in London, where she lived at the time, and a man was approaching her going in the opposite direction. As they got level the man launched himself at her, picked her up bodily and threw himself and her over a garden wall and lay with her totally underneath him, pinned and unable to move. She remembers seeing what looked like lightning coming down the road and a cacophony of noise and then it was gone. The man simply got up, brushed the pair of them off and sent her on her way. The lightning had been a German bomber strafing the road and this Good Samaritan had saved her life.

On one particular occasion that I saw my favourite duo, Chaucer had suddenly developed a very swollen and extremely painful-looking set of testicles; even the strongest man would have winced at the very sight of them. He had a testicular torsion and the huge gonad was swelling uncontrollably and stretching the scrotum to breaking point. Yes. Ouch. I explained that the only option was castration and I also told Edwina the health benefits of life without testicles so she didn't worry too much about him losing his manhood. She was as unflappable as her little charge usually was and immediately agreed to whatever would be best for him. She went on to tell me that she'd never thought to have her dogs castrated because no one had ever suggested it and did admit that Gatsby had been quite a randy dog, to say the least. I agreed that many dogs found having testicles but never being allowed to use them quite frustrating, a fact which many clients never consider when they are reluctant to give them the chop. Without skipping a beat she added, 'Yes, I suppose they must get frustrated but that never bothered Gatsby. He would always climb to the top of the staircase and then, always on his favourite step, he would stop and have a wank.'

I can't remember what I was doing at the time but I remember feeling like someone had just slapped me in the face with a wet fish, it was such a shock. I'd looked up in obvious surprise at the use of the profanity from the most unlikely mouth I could have imagined and she just met my gaze with a wonderful twinkle in her eye and the slightest of smiles curling the corners of her mouth. Never mind the snippets of people's lives that *Vets in Practice* captured, Edwina's whole life story should have been made into a Hollywood epic, and several years later when she died the world definitely became a poorer place.

If you work anywhere for any length of time in a job where you deal regularly with the public, you will inevitably become attached to some of your clients, as I did to Edwina. Equally, on the rare occasions that you lose such a friend you feel a genuine sense of loss, even if you only ever saw them at the surgery. Edwina and I had become very close and ultimately I went through the death of Chaucer with her and visited her socially on numerous occasions. I have to say that I was devastated when she died but, as it turned out, she tackled death in exactly the same head-on way she had squeezed every ounce of living out of her life. When I went to her funeral I was crying before I even sat down but laughter soon came, chokingly intermingled with my tears, when I was handed the order of service. The front page was a picture of Edwina taken over a decade before her death. She had, quite before it was fashionable, ordered herself an eco-friendly cardboard coffin and, when it had arrived, she had rung her great friend of many years, John, to come and have a look at it. Apparently he had asked in an exasperated voice what would happen if it rained, having conjured up a mental picture of the box going soggy and Edwina tumbling out for all to see before she even made it to the grave. The photo that had made me smile was taken the day the coffin arrived and showed Edwina standing inside the upright box, arms reverently crossed across her chest with her biggest, cheekiest and most wickedly wonderful smile on her face. Above the photograph, in Edwina's inimitable hand and vibrant style, was written the simple sentence, 'Please try to remember the FUN times.' I still have it pinned up in the kitchen where I can see her smile and read her words to remind me that nothing should be taken for granted and life must be lived to the full. During the service her daughter, Genevieve, gave a wonderful speech and told us all that what we couldn't see underneath the flowers on top of Edwina's cardboard coffin was that she had put a sticker on it that said 'I've been everywhere.' What a rare and wonderful human being.

This kind of personal loss is thankfully rare, but something that vets must deal with pretty much on a daily basis is the loss of animals. This can affect you greatly in a number of ways, and for me it is one of the hardest aspects of the job because of the strain on the emotions. Often I am almost as devastated to have to put down an animal I have known for years as if it were mine, but equally hard to bear is how grief-stricken the owners are. I have been through this myself and the feelings which come with deciding when your beloved animal is going to die are something that vet school can never teach. Not only do you have to cope with all the normal stages of grief, from denial all the way through to acceptance, but there is a shocking and totally overwhelming feeling of guilt. Many owners, myself included, feel like they are signing a death warrant by asking for their animal's life to be ended. When I lost my dog, Penny, who I had had since I was eleven years old, I suddenly realised that I had made every decision through her whole life. I had decided when she ate, slept and walked, and then I was deciding when she should die, and it crushed me. I strongly believe that one of the most important parts of our job as vets is to take as much of this guilt away from owners as possible to try to ease their pain in any way we can. I've never felt able to allow another vet to make this decision for my own animals. This final act of kindness, for that is what I truly believe it to be, is the least I can do for a cherished part of my family and my life, but the pain that comes with that feels almost unbearable. This makes me all the more aware of the help my clients so often need.

That said, the fact is that there are rare occasions where animals and owners can be horrendously difficult, and sometimes downright awful, so from time to time death isn't quite as sad as it might be. If I was in any doubt that this feeling was universal among vets, a friend of mine, who was a horse vet down south when I worked in Dulverton, summed it up beautifully one day. We were away on a snowboarding holiday and he had just come down an incredible run of soft, deep, powder snow, which for many a snowboarder is a heavenly experience. He got to the bottom, whooping with joy and quite out of the blue said, 'Wow. That was better than shooting a horse you've hated for years!'

I was really shocked at the time because it was the kind of thing I suspected a lot of vets felt at one time or another but never admitted and I had to smile at his honesty. But the smile turned into unstoppable laughter when he added, quite unexpectedly, 'Which is a very close second to shooting some of their bloody owners!' Please rest assured that these owner and beast combinations are very much in the minority!

Tackling euthanasia is a huge part of our job and it is so important that it is handled the right way. It should be a smooth and beautiful way for an animal to die, but sometimes the fear of what might happen can be very stressful for a fledgling vet. I'm sure we've all heard the incredibly rare tales about humans waking up in the morgue, and new vet graduates have the same irrational fears about whether animals really are dead once the deed has been done. In my first few years it was something I always double- and triple-checked because the alternative was just too unthinkable.

When I first moved to Cheltenham I'd been qualified just over a year and was feeling more and more confident with all the aspects of my job, but, as I'm sure many vets will tell you, you can never afford to get too complacent, especially when it comes to serious matters like death. During one very manic evening surgery I knew I had a euthanasia case coming in. It's never ideal to try to wedge these in to a normal consultation slot because they need time for good communication, explanation of what will happen and plenty of time for the owner to have with the animal before and after if they need it, so I knew I was going to be up against it if I wanted it done right. When the time came I called the man in with his dog, and Ray the nurse was already on hand to help with everything we needed. The owner was in his twenties, I would guess, and brought in some kind of power tool with him and laid it on one of the chairs in the consultation room. I didn't pay much heed to it because I just assumed he was a workman who didn't want to leave tools on display in his van or car. He explained that the dog was his mum's but that she was too upset to come so he had volunteered. I explained everything we would be doing and chatted to him about his options for what to do with the body afterwards. He said they had everything ready for a home burial so they didn't need us to sort out a cremation, as most people do.

The whole process went perfectly and the lovely old dog very gently succumbed to the injection. I listened to the heart for the few moments it takes to be sure it has stopped and told the young man that the dog was gone. This was when he said he would go and get the box he'd made. He hadn't mentioned this and I'd never come across this kind of thing before so Ray and I just waited and exchanged a rather quizzical glance, wondering what would happen next. The dog wasn't particularly small and, sure enough, the young man soon came back into the room with a large wooden, handcrafted box with a lid. He placed it on the floor and lifted the lid, and we could see that the box was beautifully lined, just like a coffin. He placed the dog carefully inside and put the lid on. Then he got what turned out to be his power screwdriver that I had so quickly dismissed when he arrived and proceeded to very efficiently and very permanently secure the dog inside. I remember watching, mesmerised, as the lid was so securely battened down and I couldn't help thinking to myself that if I had any worries about whether the dog was dead or not this time, no one was ever going to find out.

When he finished he gave us a cheery goodbye, thanked us once again and hefted the big load onto his shoulder and left. We stared after him, more than a little surprised by the whole thing, looked at each other, shrugged and chalked the experience into our brains as another notch in the spectrum of how people cope with the loss of their pet. But I hadn't seen anything yet. A couple of years later in Tewkesbury, Julie and I saw it all.

A lovely woman and her family came to us one day with a very ill and very old little dog. There was virtually nothing we could do for him except try to make him comfortable while the family came to terms with the impending loss.

Everybody grieves in different ways and by then I'd seen most reactions, ranging from apparently cold disinterest to open, heartbreaking wailing, so I thought I was pretty much prepared for anything. The owner was totally distraught, as is understandable when you lose what is to many people an integral member of the family, sometimes loved more than some of the human members! There were obviously a lot of tears when I told her that the kindest thing to do would be to put the dog to sleep and that it wasn't going to be long before that needed to be done. And in the week or so that followed we started to become aware just what the death of this beloved pet would entail.

First of all we had to take delivery of the Poffin. This is a bona fide pet coffin, just the same as but smaller than the human-sized one you might be buried in, and a great deal fancier than the cardboard box Edwina had chosen. The Poffin was delivered to the surgery and it certainly was beautiful. It was a perfect miniature coffin with carvings, handles and a padded purple satin lining.

After we had put the dog to sleep we kept him at the surgery until the owner had made the final preparations. We were not to close the coffin lid until she had come to the surgery with a poem she had written that was to go into the coffin with the dog. Julie and I waited for her to arrive so we could complete our part of the process. The owner didn't want to see the dog, which is a completely normal reaction, so she handed over the poem and a flower to go with it and we went away to the prep room to perform our first such funeral ritual. We very gently placed the dog and his poem and flower into the coffin and arranged him so he looked comfortable. It may sound silly but this is something I always try to do after death. Then we closed the lid firmly into place and were about to carry him out to his owner when we looked at each other across the lid and obviously both had the same thought at the same time: how on earth were we supposed to carry his coffin? The whole thing was so surreal and so like an actual human funeral that we suddenly realised we were like pall-bearers. Were we supposed to hoist the ensemble sombrely aloft and carry it out on our shoulders while some sad music played eerily through the practice? Suddenly, I have to confess, the whole thing struck us as quite funny in that way that the saddest of times sometimes can and we needed a few moments to compose ourselves. Eventually we simply decided to carry the coffin between us normally and hand him over before anything could start to go wrong.

With our part done, the woman left to go to the local pet crematorium where she was planning to wait while he and his coffin were cremated, and then to collect his ashes and take them home for the final part of the plan. This involved the local vicar coming to do a special blessing of the ashes before they were placed in a commemorative stone in the garden. Whatever your views on what pets mean to different people, stories like this have proved to me over the years that we must all cope with such a loss in our own way and that it is not our place to judge others. What other cases have taught me is that plans for the event of death are not always so regimented, detailed or thought through to anything like this level.

Graham, a friend of mine, is a sound man I have worked with for a few years now on various filming escapades. One of the brilliant things about television crews is their breadth of experience of people from all walks of life and the calamities that befall them. They always have brilliant stories and one of his is an all-time favourite of mine. He and his girlfriend were dog- and house-sitting for a friend in an area of London across town from where they lived. As is so often the case, in my experience, the dog decided that his owners being away was the perfect time to pop his clogs and land someone else well and truly up the creek without a paddle. Graham was away filming and unreachable and his girlfriend, Lou, wasn't really sure what to do so she decided she would ring the local vet to get some advice. They advised her to bring the dog in and they could then keep its body properly stored until the owners came back from their holiday and could decide what they wanted to do about cremation or burial.

Living in London, Lou didn't have a car and the thought of trying to get a taxi to take her and a dead dog across town didn't seem like it was going to work, so she decided to take the body in a large suitcase on the tube. The dog was a Labrador, not too big, but still quite a tricky proposition for a slightly built young woman to get from one place to another with ease.

As she approached the set of turnstiles she hauled and heaved the suitcase to go through the barriers at which point a very chivalrous young man approached her and asked if he could help her with her bag. She was really relieved and readily accepted the offer. As he picked it up with some difficulty, he exclaimed at the weight and asked her what she had in there. Obviously not wanting to tell him it was a dead dog, Lou smiled and told him it was just a load of DVDs and things she was moving between flats. It was at this point the man, who apparently was not all that chivalrous after all, hoicked the suitcase onto his shoulder and legged it, obviously proud of the fact that he'd struck gold with his well-practised scam of feigning help. How I would have loved to have been a fly on the wall when the cheeky thieving weasel opened the bag to inspect his haul only to find a gently rotting dog inside. Divine justice? I believe so.

It's not just thieves who sometimes come across death when they least expect it either. My friend Dan is a vet who's very chilled out, very experienced and has seen most things during his time. He has a relaxed and philosophical outlook on life and when you combine that with his wonderful, lilting Scottish accent you have a cracker of a colleague who can always make you smile when you're feeling a little overwhelmed and who can always put life into perspective for you.

Dan had to do a house visit one day to put a dog to sleep for a long-standing client. The second-floor flat was in a narrow road and he'd had to park a couple of streets away because the spaces were so limited. The euthanasia had gone beautifully smoothly and he said his goodbyes and carried the dog away in his arms to be cremated. When he got out of the flat and down the stairs he knew it wouldn't look very nice to carry the dead dog the few roads to his car so he got a body bag, which happened to be bright pink, out of his visit box and gently slid the dog inside. He held the top together in one hand and his box in the other and left the flat, heading for the zebra crossing just up the street near the corner. He was halfway over the crossing as a car came round the corner a little too quickly and slammed on the brakes at the sight of him. As luck or fate would have it, this was the exact same moment that the bag split and the dog came tumbling out to lie inert at Dan's feet on the road.

All the horrified driver saw was the recumbent and motionless animal: he hadn't seen the bag break. He leapt from the car and ran round to the front of the bonnet, staring in shock and disbelief at the body. 'Oh my God!' he cried, clamping his hands over his head and looking at Dan with horror, 'I'm *so* sorry. I didn't even see your dog.'

'Och, that's all right,' Dan replied, scooping the dog off the road and tucking him under his arm, 'he was dead already.' He sauntered off happily across the road, leaving the poor man gaping after him, no doubt wondering what on earth possessed this madman to wander the streets with his dead pet.

It was after we had moved to Cheltenham that I got the opportunity to do some actual television presenting. All the time we were on *Vets In Practice* we were merely subjects, constantly reminded not to look at the camera under any circumstances. At the same time our regional ITV channel had a popular programme called *Heart of the Country* and they were making an offshoot called *Heart of the Country Goes Wild*, all about British wildlife and some of the more exotic types of pets. I was really keen to be involved because it sounded like fascinating work. Not only would I get some time out of the surgery and meet some interesting people, but I'd also get to see some animals that I hadn't encountered before. I was petrified about talking to camera and being a proper presenter, but the interest overtook the fear and I readily agreed. From then on I realised that television takes the quirky nature of people you encounter every day and distils it until the researchers have found the most interesting or, to put it another way, barking mad, members of society.

My first day working on the show was an episode about ferrets. We do come across ferrets quite commonly at the surgery and there are many ferrets kept as working animals as well as pets. We were going to be filming in a small town which had a dedicated ferret pet shop; the town's annual festival also featured the hotly contested ferret-racing championship. Being from the Medway Towns, where the keeping of ferrets is about as common as a 4 x 4 driver pulling over to let you past on a narrow country lane, this all seemed a bit odd but I was intrigued to know what the ferret-fanatic fraternity was all about.

We started easily enough with some shots of me walking through the festivities and then we went to the pet shop to see their specialist ferret paraphernalia and meet some of the clientele. This was when the day started to go downhill for me and my very strong belief that animals should be left alone as much as possible and treated like animals, not humans, babies or dolls. The shop had a whole section devoted to clothes which you could dress your ferret up in. Understand that this wasn't to keep ferrets warm or to provide protection while they were down holes killing innocent wildlife their owners didn't like, because on the whole ferrets are pretty well designed to cope with the jobs and lifestyle they evolved for. This was a fancy dress shop and it did a roaring trade. We were shown around and told that the Santa outfits were very popular but that the Harley Davidson leathers with matching caps were the best sellers. I found myself scouring the shelves to see if there were any Indian brave outfits or policeman costumes on the off chance that if someone had six ferrets they could make themselves a little Village People tribute act. Are ferrets' legs long enough to do the actions for 'YMCA', I wondered?

I was starting to feel the onset of lockjaw from all the fake smiling I was doing, and wondering if I could escape, when we had to go and film the big race. This involved some brightly coloured transparent tubing laid out in the street, which a large crowd gathered round. The proud owners would then stuff their racers in one end of the tube and whichever one wasn't too petrified by the whole ordeal to make it to the other end first was held aloft for the cheering masses to behold and the owner was given a prize. Now call me an animal welfare hardliner but this didn't seem to be in the best interests of the animals. Having always been opposed to animals being used purely for human entertainment, I was starting to become aware of an internal scream that was trying to make its way out of my lungs and into my mouth. Just when I thought I would lose the plot, the producer rescued me by taking me to interview some genuine ferret-lovers. At last we would get a glimpse into the psyche of the fond pet-owner rather than the pimp-my-ferret brigade.

We had two people to interview. One was a big, burly man who looked every part a ferret fanatic and the other was a woman who owned more than fifty. I tried to banish the words 'mad' and 'hoarder' from my head, in case they crept their way into the interview and ended my presenting career before it had begun, and we got stuck in. Surely I couldn't mess this up. All I had to do was ask the few simple questions the director had given me. One such question he really wanted me to tackle was the issue of the smell. Most people who've encountered ferrets at close quarters will be aware that they can be a 'bit whiffy'. Indeed, most of the ones I'd dealt with at the surgery had made me want to shower quicker than a consultation with Dave and Duke ever did, so the thought of having more than fifty of the critters living in your house left me mystified. The interview was going well and I put on my best conspiratorial, jovial smile and said to the mad hoarder, sorry, loving owner, 'But what about the smell? You've got to admit that most people would agree that they are a bit smelly?'

'Oh, it's OK,' she replied, 'I've got no sense of smell.'

'Ha ha,' I ad-libbed, 'is that because your nose is numb from having so many?'

'No,' came the reply, 'it's from a head injury when I was a child.'

There was a short pause while, in my head, a bell tolled and some tumbleweed blew past. I wasn't really sure what the answer to that was and, seeing as both my feet were firmly in my mouth, I opted for silence and waited for the director to save me by shouting 'cut'. Mental note to self: no ad-libbing if I got asked to do any more programmes. Luckily for me the woman in question didn't seem to mind my genuine mistake and took it in a very good-natured way.

At least it was only my pride that was hurt by this embarrassment. When I started doing some presenting for BBC's *Inside Out* programme it seemed that Andy, the director, was hell-bent on getting me maimed by the animals we were trying to film.

It started with parrots. We were making a film about the awful trade in illegally imported wild parrots being sold as pets into a life of abject fear and misery. Our subject was a brilliant woman who has done wonders for parrots and all sorts of birds. Bizarrely, this tiny slip of an animal crusader also ran a male escort and stripper agency. I suppose the feathers must come in handy... Anyway, as pathetic as it may sound, I got savaged on the finger by a huge bird with a vice-like beak which mistook my finger for the very small seed the woman had told me to give it. I did try to be brave and managed not to cry, but it felt like someone had shut my hand in a car door. This soon paled into insignificance, however, when we went to shoot a programme about illegally imported venomous snakes.

We went to interview a snake expert at his house and talk about the highly dangerous and very threatening trade in these deadly animals. I'm not fazed by animals on the whole and have handled snakes on numerous occasions, so I wasn't feeling worried in the slightest when Andy said he wanted us both holding one of the man's rescue snakes for the interview. Our interviewee, Ben, had a large python coiled loosely on his lap and I had a very beautiful little corn snake which kept my presenting skills tested to the limit by trying to disappear down my cleavage all the way through the interview. All went very smoothly and soon enough the animals were happily back in their enclosures, which was when Ben announced he had a spitting cobra for us to film if we wanted to because, after all, it was the venomous snake trade we were talking about.

Phil, the cameraman, who had already admitted he was totally terrified of snakes, Ben and I all trooped into the small kitchen and Phil set up his tripod. Andy retreated to the living room because of space constraints. Ben produced a large sack and got a special hook ready which is used for controlling snakes and, when we were all ready, he undid the sack and made to let the snake out slowly so that he could get hold of the tail and control the body and head with his hook. Well, this was when I realised that all the snakes I'd come across before were the slow, large, constricting type or the small and inoffensive type. This thing came out of the bag like the proverbial rat up a drainpipe at a speed I'd never seen before. Ben made a grab for it but missed and it came straight for me. Like a character from a *Tom and Jerry* cartoon I did a startled, backward leap onto the kitchen worktop with my hair standing on end, at which point the creature turned sharply ninety degrees and made straight for Phil.

Amazingly, he tracked the snake's movements with his camera as calmly as anything I've seen and didn't move a muscle when it was at the hem of his own trouser leg, winding round his boot and looking for all the world like it was about to go up his inner thigh and put an end to his baby-making prospects. By this time an apoplectic Andy was leaping up and down in the front room, shouting directions and no doubt imagining the health and safety paperwork nightmare that was going to result from a dead presenter and cameraman. In the blink of an eye, though, Ben had leapt on the cobra and had it under control. Once the adrenalin had started to subside, I realised I was still perched on the kitchen cabinets like an idiot meerkat. I clambered down as we all started laughing and breathed a sigh of relief. Phil, who should have been the most terrified of us all, still looked as cool as a cucumber and I asked him how he'd managed to stay so calm. He told me that when he's looking through the camera he has this weird kind of detachment where what he sees through the lens is happening totally separately from him. The look on his face was a picture when he watched the footage back and realised it was indeed his own foot that the demonic viper had been wound round just minutes before.

That was our close call for that particular shoot but another one of our interviewees told us about someone who hadn't been so lucky. We spent some time with a reptile expert whose job it was to assist the public and the police with dangerous snakes and other such exotic animals. If the police were called to an incident involving one of these animals they would call our man, Steve, to get the animal – and keep the officers – out of harm's way. It wasn't always venomous snakes he went to, though, as constrictors are just as capable of posing a problem. Personally, I don't agree with reptiles and exotics being kept as pets at all but his best story was one of magnificent divine retribution which proved that, in the grand scheme of things, nature usually gets the better of man.

Snakes, he said, cannot tolerate the smell of alcohol. It drives them into a frenzy. On this occasion he was called out late one night to help with someone who owned a large python.

Apparently the man had been to the pub with his mates and had had a few too many to retain good sense. He'd gone home and decided it would be a great idea to get the snake out to do whatever it is that people who own snakes do with them. He'd reached in and got his dozy, placid-looking, six-foot 'pet' out for a cuddle when disaster struck. The snake, roused from its happy slumber, took one whiff of his offensive beer breath and reacted as many a girlfriend or wife would at the fumbling advances of a drunken partner. It went for him in no uncertain terms by latching onto his whole hand.

Pythons are constrictors so don't have particularly damaging teeth but they are very good at ingesting very large items via what appears to be a rather small mouth. As the poor drunken idiot watched his arm disappearing into his pet, his booze-addled brain decided there was only one course of action available to him and he ran to the kitchen, hauling the huge snake behind him, to get the biggest, sharpest knife he could find.

This sounds like a drastic measure, I know, and you start to wince at the thought of the poor defenceless creature about to be chopped to pieces for simply reacting in the most natural way to what it perceived as a threat. But fear not, because the no-loss-to-the-gene-pool owner then started trying to cut off his own arm rather than actually trying to kill the snake. By the time the police and Steve arrived the house looked like a scene from a horror film, with blood sprayed up the walls, a determined and intact snake and a large, inebriated moron attached to it with a badly damaged right arm. Steve gently, calmly and, I suspect most importantly, soberly, removed the snake and confiscated it while the police tackled the harder part of the job in trying to get his owner some medical attention. What he probably needed most was a lobotomy and a lifetime in a secure facility where he and others would be protected from his stupidity.

It's stories like this, and the characters involved in them, that made the television work so much fun and a welcome bit of light-hearted relief from veterinary work, which can be surprisingly often very emotional and very stressful. But I also gradually realised that the television work was starting to be light relief from an increasingly disintegrating relationship.

Joe and I had been together for five years when I decided I couldn't lie to myself anymore. We'd been trying to make it work and it was no one's fault, but we just weren't well suited. As the years went by the cracks in our relationship got wider and I became more and more unhappy. We were making plans to open a practice together and as the legal side got closer and closer to completion, it became the straw that broke the camel's back. As crazy as it might sound, I knew this legal contract binding us together would be a lot harder to free myself from than the contract of marriage. The imminent approach of another 'I do' clarified my thoughts and feelings and I finally knew it was all over. Instead of embarking on an exciting new venture together I ended up being the one who walked away. It was an awful few months, which anyone who's been through something similar will understand, added to which we had what felt like a nation of devoted followers watching our every move and I felt like we'd somehow let them down, as well as failing ourselves and our families. Till death us do part? It appeared not, and I found myself once again about to move on, but this time alone and unsure about what the future might hold.

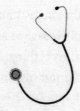

Chapter 9

There's now't as queer as folk

Joe and I were very lucky in many respects and I believe it is always best whenever possible to try not to dwell on the negatives. We'd had some great years, lots of laughter and love, and at least we didn't have children to make our decision any more complicated than it already was. As things came to their natural end I did find myself at the lowest point of my life, though. I felt like I was standing on the edge of a cliff. On the clifftop was my marriage, life, house, pets, security and the easy option to stay, but as time went by I knew I was going to jump. I was scared out of my wits but when the time came and I left all that behind, I felt like a huge weight had been lifted from my shoulders. I knew we'd both get through it somehow and the fact that Joe is very happily married with wonderful children now proves it was the right thing to do. So what of me?

Although the job at Folly Gardens had been a good move for me at the time, as things had gone wrong in my relationship with Joe I found it had a huge knock-on effect into the other areas of my life, and when we split up I realised I felt desperately unhappy with everything, work included. There wasn't just one thing I could put my finger on but the job had started to leave me cold. I suppose I was simply drained and overwhelmed. My personal life had come crashing down and, after three jobs which just hadn't been *quite right*, I suddenly felt like the career I'd striven my whole life to do had failed me too.

I made the decision to leave my job at the same time and have some time off to try to make sense of it all and hopefully regain some perspective. It was all very sudden. Joe and I were again very lucky in that we managed to sell our house very quickly. I had some money left over from the sale, which gave me some breathing space to try to figure out what I would do next.

The five animals and I moved in with my sister who also lived in Cheltenham. She had a tiny house and it took some adjusting to, but it was right next to a park so the boys were happy and the cats had a good space to roam around outside the house. But now I was really stuck and in a quandary about what I was going to do. I had wanted to be a vet for as long as I could remember and had never ever considered any other career. I had a great science degree but if general practice had not lived up to my expectations what else could I do which would fulfil my passion to work with animals, let me take my dogs to work and also pay the mortgage? I considered moving to London to work for one of the big charities but soon realised I'd hate living there. I thought about being a rep for a food or drug company but I didn't feel that it would let me make the difference to animals' lives that I'd always envisaged. Added to which, I would never leave the boys at home all day and it wouldn't be fair to them to spend so many hours in a car. I even wondered about trying to get into television work but I was nowhere near famous enough to do it the way Trude had done. So I felt well and truly stuck.

I'd been out of work for about four months when I got a phone call from Julie. When Joe and I had been planning to open our own practice we were all ready to give the job of head nurse to Julie and when everything had come to a very sudden end I really felt I'd let her down. Stoical as ever, she had shrugged it off and kept her eye out for other jobs because she too felt it was time to move on. She'd asked me for a reference for a job at a new practice that was opening up in Cheltenham and I'd gladly tried to give her the most glowing reference I could muster to make sure my failed business plans didn't keep her out of work. When she phoned it was because her new boss, Alison, was wondering if I was still unemployed and would like some part-time work. She asked Julie to give me her number and there was the offer of a casual chat if I felt like it, with no obligation.

I really needed to get back to work, not just because of money but because after a few months I realised, reassuringly, that I was really missing it. Maybe I hadn't made the wrong choice of career but had just been unlucky in my choices of job. After all, being a vet was what I had worked my whole life to do. I rang Alison and it wasn't until we started speaking that I realised how many things I wasn't prepared to put up with after my first three jobs. It became clear to me that there were practice policies in each place that I hadn't felt entirely comfortable with, but that I hadn't felt I could do anything about as a fairly recent graduate. I suddenly and refreshingly found that I had a backbone. Over the telephone I told Alison I would not condone things like tail docking and I certainly wouldn't work in a practice that performed it, I didn't want to hide my views on welfare issues like hunting and breeding and I wanted to be valued at work. Articulating the disappointment I'd felt since qualifying was like a form of therapy. Explaining it to someone else helped me get it all straight in my own head and suddenly it all became clear.

Talking to Alison was like a breath of fresh air. She was open and honest and, to my absolute joy, agreed with me about all the things I felt so passionately about. We spoke for almost an hour and I arranged to go to see the practice and meet her in person the following week so we could both decide if our initial reactions about each other were right. The practice was still in the process of being finished and was being converted from the basement of her home. Alison showed me around and Julie was there too, already starting to get involved in practice decisions even before the doors opened to the clients.

Alison knew Julie and I were close friends who had worked together for years, so she knew she was getting a ready-made team that worked. She'd also been out of clinical work for a few years so was eager for us to help with a lot of the buying decisions about drugs and equipment, or at least be involved with those decisions. I knew I'd found the job I'd been looking for. Suddenly I realised my view of my career had been skewed by a combination of bad circumstances and bad luck. I'd always been envious of people like Mike, a friend from vet school with a laugh that was so outrageously wicked and contagious it would make the devil blush without quite knowing why. He had been lucky enough to find a great job straight from university and was still there a decade later. It had always seemed inconceivable to me, but now I'd gone from rock bottom to cloud nine and I couldn't have been happier.

The practice was brand new so we all felt a sense of building it together. The success or failure of the business was going to be totally down to us. Having a female boss was also a novelty for me and I wondered if that's what felt so different. The whole atmosphere seemed gentler and more nurturing than anywhere I'd worked before; I felt valued and respected as a person and I was working in a place where the animals always came first. Best of all, it was enjoyable again. Julie and I had a great working relationship already but Alison was fun too. The emotional, mental and physical strains of the job are so great that you have to have a lighter side to stay sane and finally I'd found the perfect combination of everything I never knew I wanted until I found it. I realised I'd been so desperate to be a vet and get started that I'd gradually lost sight of all the reasons why. *This* was the career I had wanted since I was bandaging stuffed dogs at the age of six. I couldn't believe my luck.

Of course the first few weeks were slow, because we hadn't built up a large client base yet, but there was an air of excited anticipation every time the phone rang. Each new client who registered gave us a sense of achievement. As our reputation grew by word of mouth it made everyone feel so positive because we were gaining business by virtue of the fact that we were trusted. It was something we could all be really proud of. As time went by we settled into our new surroundings and suddenly I found myself in a thriving practice that I really loved.

After morning surgery one day, still in the early months, I was enjoying a guilty, leisurely cup of tea when I heard the front door go and assumed someone had come in to buy some food or make an appointment, when I heard a man's voice ask Julie if there was any chance he could see a vet, apologising profusely for just walking in off the street with no appointment. I jumped up to go and see what was wrong, assuming that he had an animal with him in need of emergency treatment, and was a little shocked when I got to the waiting room to find him all alone. I smiled, slightly relieved I wasn't going to have to reassemble the result of some horrific accident, and asked what I could do for him. He looked a bit sheepish and reached into his pocket and pulled out a small piece of tissue which he then very carefully unwrapped. He presented me with a folded-over piece of Sellotape with some strands of hair stuck in the middle of it.

'I've just got these off my daughter's head and I wondered if you could tell me what they are,' he said, his cheeks reddening ever so slightly as if he'd just admitted his house was unclean and should immediately have a large warning cross painted on the front door.

I love this sort of unexpected challenge about the job, so I gladly took the piece of sticky tape and beckoned him to follow me through to where we keep the microscope. I didn't have children at the time but I was one once and have very vivid memories of the lovely soothing sensation of the 'nit nurse' combing carefully through your hair, so I was pretty sure what we were going to see. Having said that, in hindsight, the lovely soothing sensation was followed on one occasion by weeks of being doused in hideous-smelling shampoo because the nit nurse always gets her man (or nit) and we'd been had. (The fact that parents always try to tell you that nits only like to live in clean hair never really cuts it when you're seven, though, does it!)

I focussed the microscope on the hairs and their recently-moved-in residents and smiled the satisfied smile I always get when I find parasites to look at under magnification. It may seem a small thing to get excited about but showing clients things that they never normally get to see up close is wonderful. Most parasites look monstrous under the microscope and the very normal and common head lice from his daughter's head were no exception. With their enormous legs and pointy, alien-like, dangerous-looking mouth parts, as I stepped aside for him to have a look, I eagerly anticipated the inevitable disgusted sounds and he didn't disappoint. After all the exclamations of 'Yuk' I felt suitably satisfied and had one more look myself before asking if we could keep the offending critters to add to our collection of nasties to show people. Strangely enough, he had no desire to take them home and went on his way straight to the nearest pharmacy to embark on another child's torture and, no doubt, to repeat what I'd told him about how lice always like to live in clean hair! Well, I didn't have the heart to tell him that lice don't really care about the state of the hair they inhabit, and I was sure he would want to tell his daughter and the rest of his family the usual lie, and so the myth is perpetuated...

One of my favourite all-time parasite stories happened to a vet friend of mine. With the best will in the world, vets' surgeries are to animals what doctors' surgeries are to humans; places where delightful and varied bugs can share bodies like car keys at a swingers' party. How many times have you sat in a doctor's waiting room, listened in horror to the coughing and wheezing, and known with certainty that a week later you'd have a new cold? Of course we try to keep it to a minimum, but with lots of animals in close contact sometimes it is simply inevitable that infection spreads.

My friend Sam had been a little upset when their client, the local vicar, had complained that his dog had picked up some parasites while at the surgery. Sam was very keen to placate him, but was also keen to get to the bottom of it to try to avoid it happening again in the future. The odd flea can easily travel around the place but it sounded like his dog had got something that required closer contact. She wanted to make sure that the practice protocols to prevent such things were well in place and actually working. She asked the disgruntled man of the cloth to bring in some of the parasites so that they could see what they were, find out where they had come from and offer treatment to appease their valued customer. The trouble was that the things he brought in were not recognised by anyone in the practice as normal parasites of pets so they told him that they were pretty sure they hadn't come from their surgery and suggested that he might be directing his anger in the wrong direction. He didn't take kindly to this and, because Sam still wanted to help if she could, she offered to send them away for analysis so they could be sure what they were dealing with and hopefully prove to him that they were not domestic-animal parasites and that the dog had most likely picked them up on a walk through some of the local farmland perhaps, and not at the pristine surgery. He grudgingly agreed, as long as he wasn't charged for the analysis; Sam deferred and said the practice would foot the bill. Guilty, apparently, until proven innocent. It took about a week to get the lab results back and the ensuing phone call was one that Sam cringed to make and deeply cherished at the same time. The vicar was very quiet after that, never made any more complaints about the practice, and was always as nice as pie to everyone who worked there. The parasites were human pubic lice.

Of course, as time went by and we got busier and busier, we started to gather a few great characters of our own. One of my favourite clients was a wonderful elderly woman with long, wild grey hair and a wickedly cheeky smile. She had a very sweet sausage dog called Dotty the Dachshund, who always travelled in style and arrived in a pull-along shopping trolley with her little head and two front paws poking out of the zipped top. Dotty came fairly regularly to have her nails trimmed, probably because she never walked anywhere as far as we could make out.

Her owner always loved a good natter and we could usually oblige because another brilliant perk for us was having twenty-minute appointments, which are a gold-dust rarity in veterinary practice. Twenty minutes is fantastic for thorough history-taking, treatment and, probably most importantly, good communication with clients. For short jobs like toenail clipping it was a real luxury, a chance to get to know clients through a good chinwag and, in the case of Dotty's owner, for her to tell us all about her own ailments. After a few months I was getting used to the regular updates on which joints were being worst affected by arthritis at that particular time, but as our client-vet bond grew I was once again reminded that people consider us to be priest-doctor hybrids.

Dotty's owner came in to the consulting room one day and we'd barely dispensed with the formalities before she told me she'd finally had to have something done to her knee. My reply hadn't even formed in my mouth when she unceremoniously hoisted her long skirt right to the middle of her thigh and very proudly displayed her hugely swollen post-surgical knee. As memories of the tick in the fleshy armpit came flooding back from the corner of my brain to where I'd tried to banish them, I was paralysed by the shock and also by the sight of the purple joint, barely covered in a fraying and grey bandage. There were bulges of blackish flesh poking over the tops of the bandage and, as my gaze met hers and I tried without success to close my mouth, I saw that she was wildly grinning because she was so pleased with it... She obviously saw by the unhidden mask of horror I was wearing that I couldn't have appreciated how great the knee looked so she hopped her weight onto the other foot and hoicked the skirt all the way up to facilitate a better view of the other knee, presumably for comparison.

'B-b-brilliant,' I stammered, hoping that I sounded more sincere than it sounded in my head.

'I know,' she beamed, 'look at the difference, it's amazing.'

Once again it was obvious to me that my gore threshold is way higher when it comes to animals than humans. As usual I didn't have time to ponder why this should be as I stared at the joints in question like a car crash that I couldn't look away from. To my mind, the amazing difference between the knees was that the one which had been operated on was four times the size of the other one. I finally realised that the only way to get her to cover the offending appendages back up was to tell her how superb they looked and try as swiftly as possible to divert the attention back onto Dotty and her slightly overlong nails.

The only flaw in my plan became obvious the next time I saw her. I had clearly crossed the line from politely interested vet to person of some medical training who is willing to examine and offer comment on human anatomical deformities. Because a few weeks later she brought her middle-aged son with her.

I welcomed them in, unknowingly and naively, and expected him to remain a bystander, until, that is, the opening gambit came, 'Go on, Bobby, show it to her.' Oh dear God, no. I panicked. What on earth was he going to get out? I suddenly became aware that I was trapped in an 8 foot by 8 foot basement cell with bars on the windows and one door, which was being blocked by a well-meaning but slightly maniacal old lady and a man with something so spectacularly wrong somewhere that it was apparently worthy of showing to strangers. My heart was racing and I started sweating as I hoped beyond hope that his hands didn't reach for his flies but to my eternal relief he turned round and pulled his jumper and shirt up one-handed as far as they would go.

'He's got this weird lump on his shoulder blade,' she said and then added in a voice that was half disappointment and half scolding of her son, 'Oh, you can't see it like that.' And then to me, 'You'll have to feel it.'

I tried desperately to suppress the urge to shout 'Uuuuurrrrgghhh, NO!' but had no choice but to step forward and slide one hand up inside his clammy shirt so that I could find the lump and 'have a good feel'. Of course, I didn't have a bloody clue what to say once I'd felt the thing except that he should probably get a doctor to look at it, but, luckily for me, just the fact that I'd shown an interest seemed enough to keep Dotty's slightly dotty owner as happy as she always was.

I suppose the fact is that general practice is a double-edged sword, in which the challenge and excitement of not knowing what will come through the door next is that you never know what on earth is going to come through the door next! A few months after I'd started to get over the nightmares about the shoulder lump I saw a very poorly dog called Nipper.

Nipper was a young terrier type, into everything, bum in the air, head in a hole and usually the life and soul of any party, but when he came to see me he looked dreadful. He was vomiting, jaundiced and so lethargic that he just hunched on the tabletop looking desperately miserable. He had to be admitted, of that there was no doubt. I put him straight on a drip and took bloods to try to find out why he was the colour of a certain road in the land of Oz. I had one big worry after talking to his owner and that was that he was unvaccinated. I know I've already used up my 'if you only take one thing away from this book' joker with the advice about not playing with sticks, but I think this is even more important, so here I go again. If you only take one thing away from this book it should be 'VACCINATE YOUR ANIMALS'. Don't listen to the loons who say it's all nonsense, don't use homeopathic vaccines, don't believe vets only do them to make money and don't believe that the diseases aren't around. The diseases are here and they kill and they're preventable. Rant over.

Nipper looked for all the world like a dog with leptospirosis. This is a horrible disease and it causes a variety of things depending on the strain, including organ failure, uncontrolled bleeding, liver damage and death. Nipper's bloods showed he already had damage to his liver and his yellow colour was probably a combination of blood breakdown and liver failure. We started him on very aggressive antibiotics, fluids and medication to try to alleviate his nausea. He was dangerously weak. Within two days the bloods we sent away confirmed he had lepto. Rarely, some dogs can recover from this with nursing, but it was not to be for Nipper and after a few days he finally lost his battle despite everything we had tried to do. We were all devastated. But things were about to get very odd.

As vets we have a duty to warn owners about diseases they might get from their animals. There are actually quite a lot of these, most of them minor inconveniences like scabies or other mites, but some things like psittacosis (from birds) and leptospirosis can be much more serious. It's pretty rare to get these things so please don't immediately jettison every living thing from your house besides your husband and kids (or maybe just your kids), but I felt I should warn Nipper's owners that it was a possibility, so they would know what they should be looking out for. They also had another two unvaccinated dogs so we had to get them in to be examined and get them vaccinated as soon as possible. I broached the subject as carefully as I could. I tried to be informative without scaremongering and to keep it all in perspective as best I could. The other dogs were way more at risk than the owners, a healthy, middle-aged couple whose kids had left home. I'd only ever seen the husband, not the wife, so I was relying on him to deliver this information to any other family members that had been in contact with the dog. And that was my big mistake.

The very next day the wife was in, petrified that the whole family was going to die. We had a long chat about how unlikely it was that they would have contracted anything, especially now as Nipper had first caught the disease some time before and none of the dogs or humans had been poorly at all. She seemed to be placated and left.

But within a couple of days she was back on the phone. She had been to the doctor because she was still worried and he had told her she didn't have any symptoms of lepto. Just as I had done. He had had a long chat with her about how unlikely it was. Having been told this by two medically trained professionals she was still unconvinced so she had then set off to the local hospital to demand that she be tested for leptospirosis. They had (quite sensibly) refused and that was why she was back on the phone to me. She wanted us to ring the hospital, explain about Nipper and his diagnosis and tell them they should be blood testing the whole family. I tried as much as I could to make her see that they and the doctor really knew best and once again started to stress that it was, by now, virtually impossible for her to have the disease without having had any signs at all, and that there really was no need to worry. I was seriously starting to wish I'd just taken the easy option of never mentioning it, but you can bet your life that if I hadn't, one of them would have got it and I really would have been up the creek without a paddle for NOT telling them. My only consolation was that I was part-time and wasn't in for the next couple of days. I slunk off home that night like a coward running from a fight and hoped it would have all gone away by the next week. Ha ha. No chance.

I got to work on Monday and Alison popped down from the house above to tell me about any cases she needed to hand over to me. She'd just finished and was on her way out when she paused and said, 'Oh, by the way, I had Nipper's owner on the phone last week.' My heart sank and I groaned, 'Oh no, what now?' but even I could never have imagined what now.

The wife had rung Alison because she was now undeniably convinced that her daughter had the disease. This daughter lived away from home so it was about as likely as a random stranger in the street having got it but this time she was sure because there were actual signs. It had taken Alison a while to figure out what she meant and when she told me the story I could see why. I had told the couple that one of the possible effects of the disease was liver damage. The wife had been telling Alison that her grown daughter must have the disease because she was 'losing unexpectedly large clots this month'. It wasn't until some delicate history-taking had been done that Alison realised that she meant her daughter was having a very heavy period and they were convinced that it was her damaged liver coming away in pieces, quite anatomically impossibly through her vagina. There isn't much you can say to that. How can you have a rational discussion with someone who has conjured that scenario up?

Fortunately for me it was Alison that the wife latched on to, or ended up by fluke talking to the most, in the coming weeks. Eventually, though, the whole thing was quite incredibly resolved when, after a particularly surreal consultation in which the wife asked Alison how it was that she couldn't see the non-existent brown bugs that were hatching out of her dog and her own feet and flying away, that we found out she'd been sectioned under the Mental Health Act and that was the last we saw or heard of them.

When I was seeing practice as a student I'd heard a few tales like this, which had seemed incredible at the time and I couldn't help feeling they had been a little embellished, but after a fairly short time in practice you start to realise that any job in which you deal with the general public will have a whole spectrum of human behaviour, from normal to slightly odd and, as I'd recently found out, all the way out to clinically insane. The practice where I'd spent most of my time during the university holidays had once experienced a similar problem to ours, although not on the same scale. Their client had presented a cat to my mentor, Martin, who was a brilliant vet, and explained that she was very concerned about all the shiny green bugs that were crawling all over it. He twigged pretty quickly that the bugs were only a problem for one living soul, the one who was fabricating them in her own head, but he conscientiously and diligently did a thorough, clinical examination of the cat for any sign of disease, ill health or parasites, as he was duty-bound to do. After satisfying himself that there was indeed nothing wrong with the cat, he beamed and told her the great news that the cat was in tip-top condition and full of health and vitality. The disgruntled woman's face made it plain that this was not the news she wanted and she left with an obvious air of disappointment. As with many clients in the small world of veterinary medicine, when she tried yet another practice in the area they had phoned for a history of what had been found on Martin's examination and to see if anything had been prescribed and had ended up having a fairly frank discussion about the problem, from one professional to another.

The vet she had bounced to, it turned out, was, shall we say, less scrupulous than Martin or just wanted an easy life and had prescribed a course of harmless but fairly costly herbal tablets for the 'condition' the cat was suffering from. The owner was over the moon and, Martin learned when the owner rang to tell him how wrong he'd been, the tablets worked wonders and got rid of all the bugs, but only for a limited time, after which she would go back for some more. Lucrative if you can live with your conscience, eh?

I was still pretty astounded by the first-hand experience of our own when I was talking to a good friend from university about it one day. Pete was working in a busy practice in the suburbs of Manchester at the time and had been faced with a bit of a moral dilemma himself not long before we spoke.

They'd had what appeared to be a very normal day of operating and the whole list was going swimmingly. A very sweet little dog by the name of Misty had been in for spaying and had recovered beautifully from her short anaesthetic, had some food, been out for a wee and was eagerly awaiting her owner coming to pick her up so she could go home. When her owner arrived the nurse had gone through everything that had happened that day with the surgery and carefully explained all the post-op instructions about the wound and so on. She left the owner settling the bill and went to get Misty out of her kennel and then walked her through into the waiting room for the expected joyful reunion with her owner. Misty was ecstatic to see her owner and was wagging her tail furiously and straining at the end of her lead, but to the nurse's surprise her owner just stood there and fixed the dog and then the nurse herself with a stony glare and said, 'What have you done with my dog's head?'

'I'm sorry,' replied the nurse, 'what do you mean? We haven't had to do anything to her head. She's just been in for spaying as I just explained.'

'That isn't my dog's head. The rest of it is my dog but you've put a different head on it.'

The nurse was at a complete loss as to what to say as the conversation escalated and the woman became more and more adamant that they were trying to give her some kind of amalgamation of her own dog and someone else's. The buck was most definitely not stopping with the poor nurse and she scurried away to find Pete, who had been operating that day, and explained the whole situation. He couldn't quite believe what he was hearing and went to try to smooth things out, convinced that the nurse must be somehow mistaken about what the owner was so upset about. After about two minutes of ranting in a secluded room away from the other people in the waiting room Pete realised that the nurse was by no means mistaken and that the seemingly normal client he'd seen several times before was having some kind of major break with reality.

Eventually it became blatantly clear to him that he was going to have to think well outside the box if he was going to resolve this and he decided to take a huge gamble.

'You're right,' he said with a heavy sigh of admission, 'I'm very sorry. We wanted to do an experimental head transplant and we used your dog. I know it was wrong and we shouldn't have done it but I'll fix it for you right away and we'll get your dog's head back on as soon as we can. Do you mind coming back in a couple of hours and I'll get straight on with it now? Again, I'm extremely sorry. We definitely shouldn't have done that without asking you first.'

'Well, I should think NOT!' she angrily replied, but to his huge relief readily agreed to come back just before the end of evening surgery to give them time to 'reattach' her dog's own head.

Pete led the clearly confused and very disappointed Misty back to her kennel, gave her some more food and a fond, comradely stroke of her ears and went off to start evening surgery. Sure enough, two hours later her owner came back and Pete gingerly led the once again ecstatic dog out to meet her 'mum', desperately hoping that his gamble was going to pay off, but at the same time absolutely terrified that he could be right back to square one.

'Oh *there* you are, my little darling!' her quite clearly bonkers owner enthused as the exact same Misty of two hours previously ran into her arms and the pair exchanged some long-awaited hugs, kisses and licks. Pete inwardly sighed a huge sigh of relief and was all too happy to stand there and listen to her lecture about how what they had done was terrible, and he should really be ashamed of himself, but she was very grateful that he had admitted he was in the wrong and she was positively over the moon that it had been rectified and Misty finally had her own head back on. I couldn't believe it when he told me and I knew I would never have been that quick-thinking, or had the front to try to pull off what he had done.

After I'd spoken to him I actually felt quite relieved because my story seemed to pale into insignificance compared to that. Maybe I should just be grateful that *most* of our clients were well balanced and grounded. I went home that evening for a night on call, feeling happier with the world. Little did I realise that my night on call was about to change someone's life forever.

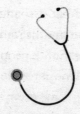

Chapter 10

What goes in doesn't always come out

It was about nine o'clock at night and I was settled happily in front of my favourite kind of escapist action film when the phone rang. The woman on the line was clearly on the verge of hysteria and it took a few moments for me to calm her down enough to get out of her what the problem was. She breathlessly told me that her dog had gone out into the garden for his night-time business and had come back in cowering and gushing blood from a wound in his groin. She had no transport and was absolutely beside herself. I grabbed a piece of paper and a pen and got her address and said I'd be there as soon as I could and in the meantime she should get a towel or something similar and try to keep as much pressure on the wound as she could.

The adrenalin was racing through my veins by the time I put the phone down and I set off at breakneck speed. Many of the 'emergency' call-outs we get are simply not emergencies in the true sense of the word but it sounded like this one might actually be a matter of life and death depending on whether or not I got there in time. Some people do overreact at the slightest bit of blood but I wasn't willing to take that chance, and also the groin area has some pretty hefty and major blood vessels running through it, so there was a chance the dog could be in serious danger of bleeding to death.

I screeched to a halt outside her door about ten minutes later and she ushered me quickly in. Her beautiful dog, Monty, was a leggy mix of what looked like collie with lurcher and as I laid him gently on his side I could see he had inherited the thin skin of the lurcher and greyhound fraternity. There was a large, ragged tear in his groin and the towel the owner had made a makeshift bandage from was already heavily stained with blood. The wound wasn't pouring but there was a steady enough ooze to make me feel the same urgency the owner had to get the dog to somewhere we could tend to him properly. It's virtually impossible to treat emergencies in the home environment, which is why vets are so often insistent on people coming in if they can.

'Right,' I said, 'we'll put him on the back seat of the car but I'm going to need you to get in beside him to keep the pressure on this wound for me, OK?' I was already gathering my car keys from the floor beside the dog as I asked the question, and I didn't really wait for a reply as I scooped the shaking and shocked dog into my arms and headed for the door. The woman, whose name I'd now learned was Sally, didn't say a word and just looked as shocked as the dog as she tried to keep step beside me and keep the towel in place as we edged our way out of the house and into the car.

We got to the surgery in minutes and Julie was already there, as I'd phoned her on the way. She had the theatre set up with everything we might need. I told Sally to stay in the waiting room while we tried to get to grips with Monty's condition and ascertain exactly what damage had been done. Julie got her a drink of water, which she really looked like she needed, and we headed off into the back of the practice to get on with our work.

I got Monty started on a drip because he was pretty pale, and because he was in quite a bit of pain I gave him a sedative combination which would give him good pain relief, reduce his anxiety and also make him pliable enough for me to get a good look at the damage. Once he was comfortable and woozy and the fluids were going nicely we eased him right onto his side and Julie gently lifted his leg up into the air and held it in place while I removed the blood-soaked towel. I clipped the scanty hair away from the area of the wound and saw with relief that the blood loss had slowed to a virtual stop, but I could see he would need surgery to repair the damage so we gave him an injection to fully anaesthetise him.

I got a bowl of warm saline and started bathing the area to get the dried blood away and get a look at the wound itself. Monty had actually been lucky in a way. Whatever he had torn himself on in the garden had been jagged and not very sharp. Tearing wounds which cut through blood vessels usually cause a wonderful survival reaction that evolution has instilled in us all called elastic recoil. Blood vessels are made of muscle, which is full of stretchy fibres, and when the vessel is torn these fibres stretch as far as they can then rebound like an elastic band, shrinking the end of the vessel into an elongated and very narrow or closed tube. This immediately helps reduce blood loss and activates the clotting mechanisms which are vital for stopping blood flow.

I parted the wound edges and could see that he certainly hadn't punctured or damaged the huge femoral artery that goes through the groin because it was pulsing away and, as it's practically the size of a drainpipe, he never would have made it to the surgery if he'd severed that. I could see the smaller vessel he'd torn and could also see that it had done its job wonderfully. All that really remained for me to do was clean the whole wound up, flush out any debris, tidy the edges to get clean ones which would heal and stitch the whole thing back together again. Because of the location and the dirty nature of the injury I placed a surgical drain in it so that we could flush it out if we needed to and to allow any fluid that might accumulate to drain out. We eased Monty into a large kennel to recover and while Julie tried to sort out the mess I'd left behind in the theatre I went to tell Sally what we'd found and that Monty was going to be fine.

We had a long chat and I made us all a cup of tea while we waited. Night-time calls have a special quality that I always cherish in some ways because of the peace and tranquillity of a place which is so often bedlam during the day. Sally went in to see Monty once he was awake and it was plain to see how much he meant to her. I told her he would need to stay in that night but should be able to go home the next day and I asked her if she'd like me to call her a cab because I needed to stay a while longer to make sure he recovered properly. Which was when she told me, to my absolute astonishment, that she hadn't left her house for the last three years because of increasingly severe agoraphobia. Until tonight.

I'd been so focussed on getting Monty to the surgery I realised I hadn't even asked her if she *could* come with me. I'd just barked instructions at her and basically frogmarched her to the car. I felt really guilty and started to apologise profusely but I soon realised she was smiling a huge smile. She said it was wonderful. She'd had to get a dog walker to take Monty for his walks since she'd got this bad and felt guilty about it. She really missed the times they'd had out together. In fact one of the reasons she'd got him in the first place was to make her get out of her house and into the world. Her forced evacuation had apparently been the wake-up call she needed and she said she felt like she could start trying again to get out on her own. She suddenly gave me a huge hug and I saw she had tears rolling down her face as well as the big smile which seemed to be a newly permanent fixture. She said that nearly losing her beloved boy had made her realise that life was too short to be locking herself away and now was the time to start to get her life back. It seemed that the time it had taken us to repair Monty had really been enough time for her to put the world to rights. Her world, at least.

She climbed into her taxi about half an hour later with a grateful smile and a small wave. I watched her face disappear out of sight with a huge mix of emotions. I'd known for a long time that my job affected a great many people in different ways because of their relationship with their animals but this was a different impact altogether and it felt truly fantastic.

I couldn't help but worry that in the morning, in the cold light of day, her adrenalin and her new resolve might have left her but at eleven o'clock sharp, as arranged, she arrived in a car with the friend who usually walked Monty. She walked in and beamed at me. Her beloved boy was back on top form and was totally ecstatic to see her. She thanked me once again way too much and off they went to start their new life together. I saw them several times in the following week or two while we finished all of Monty's post-op needs. Once his stitches had been removed and he was allowed to be released from his lead on walks, she proudly told me that she was planning a big trip up Cleeve Hill as a special celebratory first proper walk for the two of them. Cleeve Hill was a favourite of mine and the boys too and was the sort of place that blew away the cobwebs and made you feel at peace with the world, so I knew they were going to have a great time. I would have loved to have been with them, but it was clear this was something that really needed to be just the two of them, so I told her to enjoy it and said I'd wait to hear all about it next time I saw them.

As you may have gathered by now it is very often animals' owners who give us most cause to smile, laugh, cry and cringe but after about a year of working at Alison's practice we started to see a wonderful array of creatures who had no owners. A local wildlife rehabilitation centre asked us if we would take on their veterinary work and, being a relatively quiet and growing practice, we were ideally placed to do it. I was really pleased because it would be a great opportunity to see wild animals close up, and also because I would be able to help nurse some of them back to health and back into the wild where they belong. Lots of members of the public are very concerned about wildlife, as the episode of the grilled pheasant had shown, and vets are quite commonly presented with casualties to treat. As I mentioned before, if you can pick up wildlife there is a fifty-fifty chance that they will die. Nature perfectly equips animals to get away from a species which is as predatory and bloodthirsty as us humans, so they have to be very badly injured or just plain moribund to let one of us shove them in a box and drive them to a surgery.

I have to admit that soon after we started working with the centre, I did feel a little despondent because we just seemed to be putting so many animals to sleep, but Caroline, who founded and runs Vale Wildlife, had some interesting things to teach me. The first was to explain the fifty per cent thing, because she wanted to allay my fears that I was a rubbish vet. The animals they brought to us were often so badly injured that they simply expected to lose the numbers we lost. Secondly, and most importantly, she taught me that often euthanasia is the only option if an animal can't be returned to the wild absolutely one hundred per cent able to compete, otherwise you are just dooming that animal to a slow and painful death by starvation or predation. It might sound obvious to most of you but one of their biggest struggles is getting this message across to some people. They've had many cases over the years where concerned members of the public would rather, for example, a bird of prey be kept in a cage with one wing than be put to sleep. No matter what we think of death, it is certainly preferable to a life in captivity for many wild animals that would, as captives, only know fear, and be deprived of social contact and the freedom they are used to. Indeed, the wildlife work was a learning curve in lots of ways and I learnt several lessons along the way.

Lesson one – not all animals are as large as they appear. We had a lovely, shiny bank of stainless steel kennels for housing the in-patients. One particular day we had the normal couple of dogs and cats for neutering or minor ops, but we also had a very ill ferret. This was normally a working ferret but it had developed awful breathing problems and could barely move by the time we saw it. We'd X-rayed it that morning and found that it had a hugely enlarged heart which was failing, and this was causing fluid to build up in its lungs. The outlook for the poor creature was pretty grim. There are plenty of drugs we can use these days to treat dogs and cats with heart disease and some of these can be safe for ferrets, but this condition was very advanced and the finances for this working animal were simply not going to extend to palliative care. We'd given the ferret some medication to try to get some of the fluid off his chest and at least make his breathing a little less laboured while we waited for a decision from the owner about what to do. In the kennel next to his was a baby squirrel that had come in from a member of the public; it was orphaned, thin with hunger and very weak. We had given the little creature some liquid food by a tube and we would see if he could get strong enough to go to Vale to recover fully, but he was looking pretty poorly.

Later that day I had just discharged a dog and was setting about cleaning out the bowls and newspaper from his kennel when, from my crouched position, I had a level view into the ferret's cage above. He was still curled up at the back, ribcage working away, and sleeping very peacefully all things considered. My gaze was drawn to his litter tray though, as I wondered who'd thought to put a toy in there when he was clearly in no state to do any playing. Then, as my eyes adjusted to the gloom in the kennel, I thought it was a furball he'd brought up and peered in closer to see exactly what the furry foreign object in his litter tray was. As I looked closer, my brain tried to deny what my eyes were seeing as I realised with horror that it was his neighbour, the baby squirrel, and if we'd thought its days were numbered before we certainly hadn't realised that the number was one. I did a double take and immediately checked the cage next door, which was of course empty. We'd thought there was no way the creature could get through the tiny holes in the kennel door but it was obviously a lot more fur than flesh because he had undeniably escaped. How ironic that we had given the squirrel just enough energy and sustenance to make a terrific and heroic bid for freedom, while at the same time giving the ferret just enough oomph to fully relish what turned out to be his ceremonial last meal and deliver a lethal bite to his unwitting visitor. It wasn't a happy decision when the squirrel had had to plump for left or right and had chosen right. Not really survival of the fittest, by any stretch of the imagination, more like death all round and a pretty stupid-feeling vet at the end of it with some explaining to do to Vale about why they wouldn't be needing to hand rear a certain baby squirrel anytime soon.

Lesson two – despite the many experiences of footballers' and politicians' wives, not all males are unworthy cheaters. One of my favourite encounters while doing the wildlife work was with a good old-fashioned pair of common mallard ducks. Vale rang to see if they could come straight in with a casualty, a duck which had been injured on the road. Ducks, geese and swans can sometimes get easily fooled by wet roads glinting in sunshine, which look like rivers and streams from a distance. If you've ever seen the way one of these animals lands, skidding onto water, you'll wince at the thought of what happens to their feet and legs if they've picked a tarmac road by mistake. We told them to come straight down and I was a bit surprised when two ducks arrived, having only heard about one being injured.

As it transpired, it was a female who was injured and had been spotted, unable to walk, by the roadside, but when they'd gone to pick her up her boyfriend had appeared and started to get very agitated at the human intruders. Throughout the rescue attempt the male had stayed steadfastly at her side, defending her to the last. They'd actually had quite a job getting to the female, and kept having to fend off her valiant saviour until they'd managed to scoop both of them up. It hardly seemed fair to break up such a devoted couple, so in they both came, and he stayed by her throughout her treatment and recovery time with us and then on to Vale's gorgeous pond and eventually back into the wild. And the best bit of all; they'd come to us on Valentine's Day.

Lesson three – wild animals are absolutely *hooching* with parasites. Nature has a fantastic way of making sure that all animals and plants have a niche. Everything has a reason to be and, no matter how nonsensical some of them may appear to be to us, they all do something in the cycle of life. Parasites are no exception. Probably the most unfortunate species of animal I came across doing the wildlife work was the humble hedgehog. They get themselves into all sorts of scrapes, like having their legs strimmed off by overenthusiastic gardeners or being unrolled and scooped out from the inside by badgers, they are prone to infections like salmonella, and they are walking micro-zoos covered in ticks, lice and fleas. I used to feel so sorry for them but they are very robust and we helped a great many while I was there. But of course they're not the only animals to have such passengers. One afternoon a Vale volunteer had brought in a deer, which had been found trapped in a fence. This was another thing that it wasn't uncommon for us to see. Deer become spooked, run and then jump a fence only to get one leg trapped inextricably in the wire. Often by the time we saw an injured deer, it had done awful damage to the leg in trying to free itself, and this beautiful animal had been no exception. I'd examined the large deer in our consulting room where we had good space away from the dogs that were in for ops. The dogs would have been even more stressful for it than its encounter with me.

One back leg was dreadfully injured by the wire and there was a deep cut right through all the major tendons of the fetlock joint, with a very deep infection already causing disease in the joint itself. There was no option but to put the deer to sleep because the leg could not be salvaged and the animal would find captivity unbearable. I put it to sleep to end its suffering and the volunteer took it away for disposal and in no time at all it was time to start evening surgery.

After about an hour I was talking to a lovely woman and her daughter about their dog when I started to feel a tickle in my cleavage. I was wearing a scrub top I'd had on earlier but didn't think too much of it because it was the sort of sensation you get when you've got a hair trapped in your clothing, or, something that many women will relate to, in your bra. I ignored it as best I could because I thought it not very professional to shove one arm down my V-neck and have a good guddle around in my own breasts, but after a couple of minutes I became very aware of it again. Except this time it felt like something moving a tiny bit. I tried to banish the thought from my head as I tried desperately to concentrate on what I was saying. It must just be a hair. But then I had no doubts as I felt a definite scurry. Now my flesh was crawling and I needed to get the clients out as quickly as I could. I started making all the right noises and edged towards the door, eventually holding the door open and practically herding them out with a cheery wave. As soon as they'd gone I pulled the neck of my scrub top out and peered in, not really wanting to know what was going on in there. And there it was. A large flat fly, which is just what it sounds like – a big, squashed-looking, multi-legged creepy crawlie which likes to live on things like deer until they are no longer living and would then rather take up residence on anything else warm-blooded they can find – was nestled very happily in between my bosoms.

I'm not usually very squeamish about such things but the unexpected nature of it, and the sight of it just exploring in there, scurrying around in my bra, gave me one of those full-body panic reactions and I literally ran out of the consulting room, past the waiting room full of surprised-looking clients and their charges, stripping as I went, full tilt into the prep room. Julie was in there cleaning up after the day's ops and turned at the clatter of the door as a half-naked and fully hysterical vet came flying in, frantically flapping at her breasts, saying repeatedly, 'Get it off me! Get it off me!' As the tiny and totally harmless parasite was flicked full force from its comfortable new lodgings and I came to my senses, I found myself stripped to the waist in the middle of a room with a bay window looking out to the neighbours, feeling rather foolish on all kinds of levels. I sheepishly climbed into a clean scrub top, turned on my heel and steeled myself to go back and call in the next client, knowing full well that *everyone* had just witnessed the whole debacle. And so the lessons that wildlife work taught me were added to my accumulated and ever-growing experience.

Just as the flat fly had found its way into my cleavage, it turned out that the following spring was going to be the season of things ending up where they didn't belong. Our first such candidate was a very lively, eternally happy, springer spaniel, aptly called Bouncer. I heard about him before I saw him, which also turned out to be why he proved to be one of the easiest diagnoses I've ever had. He had done what so many animals I've encountered over the years had chosen to do and that was to behave perfectly reasonably until their owner had left them in someone else's care and then do something very stupid. The young woman who was friends with his actual owners, and who was looking after him with her husband while they were away for a couple of weeks, rang in a panic on day two of what was going to be a long couple of weeks by the sound of it. She and her husband had visitors in the shape of their small nieces and had bought each of them a little treat. A lovely Kinder Surprise egg. As it turned out, the surprise was that when one of the little darlings fumbled the egg out of its wrapper, her chocolate-craving, five-year-old reflexes weren't even in the same league as the finely honed skills of Bouncer, who pounced, or, more accurately, bounced on it from about two metres away with the speed and accuracy of a cheetah taking down a gazelle and swallowed it whole in a single gulp.

Claire, the young woman, had rung us straight away to see what she should do. I asked her if there was any chance at all that the egg had been crunched even a tiny bit before it went down but she just couldn't tell because it had all happened so fast. I told her that it can be very surprising how many things can make their way through an animal's digestive tract but that if there was any hint of vomiting or malaise then we should see him straight away.

Sure enough, two days later Claire was back on the phone because Bouncer was as lively as ever but had brought up his whole breakfast that day. He had to come in. As I mentioned before, X-rays can be somewhat disappointing when it comes to some foreign bodies but I had high hopes for this one. I wasn't sure how well plastic was going to show up on an X-ray but when I held the first view up to the light box there in

Bouncer's stomach, as plain as day, was the ovoid shape of the inside of a Kinder egg. And even better was that you could just about make out the shape of the little toy that was inside. This set off all the usual speculation about what exactly we might find but what there was no need to speculate about was the fact that it had to come out, because it was totally intact and there was no way it was going to pass naturally.

The surgery was actually very straightforward compared to some of these hunting expeditions. I didn't have feet and feet of intestines to trawl because the object was quite clearly in the stomach and we had a concise and unequivocal history and timeline, which is pretty rare in these cases. I clipped the fur from Bouncer's tummy, from halfway up his sternum to his pelvis, and we got him sterilised and prepped. I made my incision high up near his ribcage to get to his stomach, reached in and immediately found the big lump in the empty organ. I held it between my thumb and fingers and sliced into the stomach wall over the top of it and the little egg popped out like an egg that had just been laid. Julie was eagerly waiting with a bowl and, because I was sterile and needed to get on with the job at hand, she got the glory of being the one to open the egg and see if any of us had guessed the contents correctly. In case you were wondering, it was a sort of space monkey, which none of us had guessed, not unsurprisingly, because what on earth is a space monkey?

Anyway, as good practice dictates, I felt the full length of his intestines to make sure we hadn't missed anything else unknown he might have snaffled and, satisfied with our bounty, stitched all his layers back up again and let him wake up. It was with great pleasure the following day when Bouncer went home that I presented Claire with the little plastic bag containing the two halves of the egg and the wildly grinning and waving space monkey. Everyone likes a souvenir, don't they?

It's very weird how you can go months or even years without seeing certain conditions and then, like the proverbial London bus, three come along at once. About three weeks after we'd retrieved Bouncer's egg I encountered an equally vivacious, slightly more lunatic and somewhat less endearing boxer dog by the name of Ramone. When I opened the door of the consulting room to call his owner in, I saw a huge boxer leap from his seated position and launch his slight owner off her seat. She just managed to shout at her two kids to follow her as he dragged her into the room and promptly shoved his nose right into my groin, slobbered all over my trousers and then urinated up the leg of the consulting table. Now, if you're going take one thing away from this book... No, I won't abuse my favourite phrase but I wasn't at all surprised to glance between his muscly legs and see a large pair of testicles dangling there, which explained a lot of his unwanted behaviour straight away. After he'd urinated all over the rest of the room, still dragging his owner round every corner, snuffling and slobbering as if she wasn't even there, I asked her if she'd ever thought of having him castrated. I went on to say that it would almost certainly help with his unruly, uncontrolled and, in my humble view, antisocial (and very unpleasant, although I kept this last part to myself) behaviour. She put one final huge effort into getting hold of his collar and hauled him to a sitting position at her side as she panted for enough breath to answer my question.

'Oh no, we wouldn't want to spoil his character,' she replied. After a few seconds of stunned silence on my part, while I tried with all my might not to question whether the 'character' she was referring to was the amazing display of crotch-sniffing and inappropriate covering of my whole room in piss, I decided eventually that I would clearly be banging my head against a wall. I opted instead to enquire why she had decided to grace us with his presence that fine day.

As it turned out, they'd just registered with us because we were closer to where they lived, but she was pretty sure Ramone was up to another trick of his, which had seen him at his previous vet's for surgery on two occasions in the last year. He was a gravel eater.

This might sound odd but is actually not that uncommon. Some dogs almost certainly just end up ingesting little bits of gravel when they find something else tasty on top of it, but others, like Ramone, actually seem to seek the stuff out. Apparently Ramone wasn't quite himself that day and was a bit subdued, which left the mind boggling at how uncontrollable all 40 kilos of him must be on a good day, and he was displaying all the same signs as his last two times so his owner was pretty sure what we were going to find. He was way too bouncy and large to get a good feel of his guts so we had to admit him in order to sedate him for a good palpation and X-rays. It also gave us time to contact his old vet's for his records which, when they arrived by fax about twenty minutes later, showed the extent of his 'habit'. Both times previously he'd needed multiple incisions in several different sites throughout his intestines and stomach to remove sizeable amounts of gravel apparently snaffled from his owners' front driveway.

That day turned out to be no exception and, after not being able to feel much because of his size, we X-rayed him and saw what looked like masses of small stones scattered along the length of his small intestine and stomach. This wasn't going to be as easy or quick as Bouncer by a long chalk, and an hour and a half later I finally got him back in his kennel, having had to make seven separate incisions to get to all the pieces. Intestines need very careful suturing indeed to make sure there are no leaks and this was the most time-consuming part of the whole process. But he and I were lucky this time too, looking at the silver lining, because he had no damaged bowel, which meant he hadn't had to have any lengths of gut removed and, hopefully, was not in the most at-risk group post-surgery because of it.

When his owner came to pick him up she was already well prepared for the large bill because of her previous experiences and as she sighed and handed over her credit card she asked if I had any thoughts on how to stop him doing it. It's a good question and not one I had an easy answer to. It was the kind of question a behaviourist would spend about two hours getting a full history for and I knew I was out of my area of expertise.

'The driveway cost us a fortune about two years ago and it was something my husband had been planning for ages,' she told me.

As we spoke a few things became very clear. Firstly, her husband *loved* that driveway, secondly, they'd saved up for it for a very long time, and thirdly, it was definitely the scene of the repeated crimes because they'd seen him eating it. I thought it was time for common sense to prevail so I told her how serious it could be for Ramone to keep having intestinal surgery. I also pointed out that their vet's bills combined were probably going to start approaching what the driveway had cost them in the first place and maybe it was time to admit defeat and just have the bloody thing paved over. When Ramone came in for his post-op check his owner told me that, unbeknown to her, her husband had already rung round to get some quotes on the day of Ramone's op, apparently having weighed up whether he loved the gravel or his dog more, and Ramone had won out. If you can't keep the dog away from the gravel, you just have to take the gravel away from the dog. Sure enough, when I left the practice some time later Ramone had stayed gravel-free and surgery-free, and had probably paid for the new tarmac by staying healthy, but sadly still had his nuts, his slobber and the total lack of training to keep his nose out of my nether regions every time I saw him! You can't win them all.

I said that that summer had brought us three of these cases in quick succession, and number three was a dog endearingly called Muppet because of his perpetually gormless expression. He was a beautiful dark-yellow Labrador, the breed we most often encounter in these circumstances where appetite rules all. I'd known Muppet for a few years now because his owner, Hannah, had been one of my clients in my first job in Cheltenham and had very faithfully moved practice with me to Tewkesbury and then back to Cheltenham, which was very flattering.

Muppet's particular penchant was socks from the dirty laundry basket. He'd started as a puppy just wanting to take socks to his bed, possibly because the smell was comforting, and whenever Hannah found an odd sock in the laundry she could usually be pretty sure she would find the other badly buried in Muppet's bed or being carried round like a prize. He always looked bereft whenever she took his sock away and would sulk for ages in his bed until he managed to grab the next one.

He was about eighteen months old the first time we'd had to operate on him to actually remove a sock, and was almost three the second time his obsession went too far. As you can imagine, there were some pretty severe laundry rules put in place in the house, which was probably why it had been a while since we'd seen him but I must admit that Hannah and I had assumed he would eventually grow out of his habit, as many young dogs do. That was why I was surprised to see the pair of them on the waiting-room list with the single word 'sock' in the space on the screen for the reason why the animal was coming in.

I smiled and shook my head as Hannah came in and she gave me a very resigned smile herself. They thought they'd been so careful and she said that she was pretty sure they'd managed to keep him away from the laundry, but two days beforehand she'd found a solitary sock and that morning Muppet had started bringing up bile and was certainly off colour. He did seem very sad and wasn't his usual enthusiastic self at all as I gently felt his abdomen. Because he wasn't eating well and had been sick a few times, and also because he'd always been a beautifully lean dog, I found I could palpate his whole abdomen really well and there wasn't much to feel. The trouble is you can never be sure and with long, thin foreign bodies like socks you could easily miss something. I still felt it was worth giving him the benefit of the doubt. I gave him some medication to help with his vomiting and gave Hannah some special food for him to have to see if he just had an upset stomach, which was much more likely at his age and with his signs.

The next afternoon he was much the same so we booked him in for investigations the following day and I hoped there was a chance he would turn a corner overnight and be back to his old self by the time he came in. But that morning he was sick again and we admitted him as planned.

When he was anaesthetised and fully floppy I had another really good feel around and still came up with nothing. We X-rayed his abdomen in stages because he was a big dog and still there seemed to be nothing. Not only was there nothing obvious blocking the guts, there just wasn't any sign of an obstruction at all. No gas, no distended loops of bowel, just feet and feet of very empty-looking bowels. I was pondering the final view we'd taken and wondering whether I should plump for further medication or just bite the bullet and get in there when something caught my eye. Right in his pelvis I could just make out a slightly odd pattern on the X-ray. I knew cloth would appear the same colour as his tissues but there was just a hint of an unnatural marking in his colon which I managed to convince myself might just be the knitted pattern of a missing sock.

I grabbed a pair of rubber gloves and some KY jelly and lifted the sleeping Muppet's tail. With my finger inserted as far as it could go into his bottom, I thought I could just feel the edge of something. It was tantalisingly close. I scooped the poo out of his rectum and felt in again, this time sure I could feel something. I reached as far as I could but I just couldn't get hold of what I was becoming more and more sure was the sock. I got a pair of long tissue forceps and very gently pushed them inside. When I met resistance I opened them a tiny amount, advanced and closed them down onto the blockage. I pulled very gently because I was doing the whole thing blind and, sure enough, the thing started to move. I eased the forceps out with bated breath and was greeted by a sight that was wonderful and gross all at the same time. Covered in poo, and having been through all the juices and churning of the whole intestinal tract for some days, was a bright red something. I held it aloft like Excalibur, very proud of myself indeed, and told Julie to turn off the anaesthetic gas because Muppet was escaping the scalpel that day. I went to rinse off Hannah's souvenir but after I'd had it under the tap for a few minutes I knew the ensuing phone call wasn't going to be what either of us had imagined that morning.

'Hi, Hannah, it's Emma.'

'Oh hi, how's Muppet? Did you have to operate?'

'No, we didn't, which was a real relief, but I've got some good news and some bad news.'

'Yeeesss?' she asked hesitantly.

'Well, the bad news is that I didn't find the missing sock, so I can't help you there, but the good news is that I did find a very nice, lacy red G-string.' I grinned as I delivered the line and I could imagine from the silence that Hannah's cheeks were probably approaching the scarlet colour of her thong that I'd pulled from Muppet's backside just half an hour before!

I suppose it must have been around the end of April that I triumphantly retrieved this little piece of treasure. Spring was giving way to early signs of summer, I was having an absolute ball at work, I had lots of clients who'd become friends over the years and the practice was going brilliantly. Everything seemed perfect. It was the end of evening surgery one day when Alison popped down from upstairs and said, 'How would you like an all-expenses-paid trip to Kansas?'

Well, I wasn't going to say no, was I? Alison wanted to organise the trip for me to say thank you for everything over the first couple of years that the practice had been open. Every year a large pet-food company got together a group of vets from all over Europe and sent them first to the North American Veterinary Conference, wherever that was being held in the States, and then on to their headquarters in Topeka, Kansas for more lectures and a look round the facilities there to see first-hand how their foods are produced. Because of Alison's long-standing ties with the company she'd managed to get me a place on the trip if I wanted to go. I'd only been to the States once many years before and it sounded like too good an opportunity to turn down so I readily accepted. It was quite short notice as there were only a couple of months before I was supposed to go, so I had to decide quickly and get my flights and accommodation booked. It was all a bit of a whirlwind and it wasn't until nearer the time that I realised I would be going alone with a load of people I didn't know and, added to that, they would all be vets. This might sound like an obvious thing to say and not necessarily a problem but I realised that the wrong group of vets could make this one of the dullest trips I'd ever experience in my life. Ah well, I have my rule of never having regrets and it was all booked and paid for now. The day before I flew, I finished evening surgery and nipped upstairs to say goodbye to Alison and tell her about any cases she might see while I was away for the ten days. As I walked down the front steps and waved goodbye I turned and said, 'This could be the most boring trip imaginable, all being vets, couldn't it?'

'It could be,' she said, then added, 'in fact, when I went we got to Topeka and the first night I asked the hotel receptionist what there was to do, she replied that there wasn't much because "nuthin' ever happens in Topeka, Kansas, ma'am".' She smiled as she finished the sentence in a perfect Deep South accent and I said my goodbyes and left.

Oh, how wrong that receptionist turned out to be.

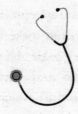

Chapter 11

It really shouldn't happen to a vet

My first stop was Charlotte, North Carolina for two days of the conference before flying to Topeka. I was a couple of days later arriving than the rest of the delegates because of flight arrangements and work commitments, and I arrived quite late in the evening so I just headed straight to bed to relax. The next day I had instructions to go to the conference centre and find the company's stand so that I could meet the organiser and the rest of the delegates. I went to a lecture first and aimed for the exhibition hall for the morning coffee break, when I was most likely to find Anne-Marie, the woman whose name I'd been given. I got there to find a bustling commercial exhibit full of very 'vetty-looking' people. There was a sea of checked shirts, chinos and cords, which didn't do much for my worries about the type of vets that might be on the course. I found Anne-Marie and she immediately put me at ease because she was jovial, relaxed and made me feel immediately welcome.

She guided me over to the edge of the stand and said I was just in time to meet a few of the other British vets. Chris and Neil were first to shake my hand and then I was introduced to a man called Mark, who shook my hand and gave me a huge, infectious, sparkling smile which made his whole face light up. And about forty-eight hours later we were hopelessly and totally in love.

Although this must sound totally slushy, I had never believed in love at first sight. I wasn't looking for it, and I certainly wasn't expecting it, but it hit me like a train and there was no getting away from it. When we met, Mark was adorned in the obligatory vet 'uniform' of chinos and a checked shirt and could easily have been mistaken for 'any other man'. Oh, hang on, apart from that smile and the fact that he was gorgeous! We headed to a lecture and then decided to go for a drink with Chris. As we stepped out of the gloom into the bright North Carolina sunshine, Mark reached into his bag and put on a pair of surf-style sunglasses. Hmm, I thought, a definite sign that he might not be as vetty as he had at first appeared. The three of us spent the afternoon together and arranged to go out for dinner later that night. Turning up to meet me that evening in fairly scruffy jeans and a T-shirt, he (probably unwittingly) became even more attractive to me. I've never been a fan of flashy designer fashion and have always found open displays of wealth through clothing and accessories somewhat off-putting. You know the type I mean – all wardrobe, no Narnia!

When we arrived at Chris's hotel he was nowhere to be found so fate played a hand and we ended up going out alone. Someone at the hotel recommended a very good restaurant called Aquavina and we set off. When we arrived they were fully booked, but, as fate seemed hell-bent on making sure we stayed together, a no-show by a couple who had reserved a table allowed us to get in for the evening. We had a beautiful meal and lovely wine in a great atmosphere and I'm sure it seemed all the more special because I was already smitten and we talked and talked as if we'd known each other forever. I didn't want the evening to end.

As the week went by we found we had a surprising amount in common, particularly our childhoods and the way we'd been brought up. We'd both been married before but neither of us had children and we had both left those relationships without regrets, but having learned from them what we did and didn't want in a partner. All this said, I simply couldn't believe that the way I felt could possibly be reciprocated because I'd never felt such strong emotions before. I was also convinced that Mark was 'way out of my league' so surely couldn't be interested beyond being friends. By the time we parted ways at the airport a few days later the fact that I thought I'd never see him again seemed to physically hurt. I went from being on an enormous high to feeling lost and devastated. But, to my complete astonishment and absolute joy, a few days after we got back to England we couldn't resist the urge to phone each other and very soon admitted how we felt.

Sadly for Alison, her exercise in bonding me to the practice backfired horribly and, three months after I'd waved goodbye to her on the front steps on my way to Kansas, I handed my notice in. Mark was a partner in a big practice in Yorkshire and, because I was only an employee, it made much more sense for me to move to his neck of the woods when it became blatantly obvious to all concerned that our 'holiday' infatuation was in fact the real thing. This was really hard to do because I genuinely loved my job there, but I've never been one who's able to ignore my emotions, especially when they're as all-consuming as they were then.

I had three months left to work before I took another leap into the unknown and my last few months were certainly not dull. One Saturday, when I was on call for the weekend, I'd finished morning surgery and, before heading home, I was sitting behind the reception desk catching up on some paperwork and putting some lab results on the computer. There was suddenly a frantic clatter at the front door and a young woman came bursting down the steps, hysterically calling for someone to help her and clutching a cat to her chest. I jumped up and ushered her into the prep room, trying to find out as we went what was wrong. She just kept sobbing that her cat was choking and couldn't breathe. I prised the beautiful tabby cat out of her arms and laid him on the table and I could immediately see that she wasn't exaggerating. The cat was trying desperately to keep himself upright, mouth gaping wide open, tongue out, clawing for air. His ribcage was heaving with the effort and he kept rolling onto his side with exhaustion and then trying to get back up to keep his airway as open as possible. There was no time to get help so I asked the owner to keep a loose hold of him while I got some things together. In his gasping and open mouth I had already seen what looked like a huge area of tissue damage to his tongue and mouth and I suspected he'd eaten or drunk something chemically caustic, which was causing a huge reaction in his throat. I put a mask attached to an oxygen cylinder as close to his face as I could without distressing him further, grabbed a small pen torch and showed his owner how to hold his head so I could get a look in his mouth. The soft tissue of the whole mouth and throat was grossly swollen and looked corroded with huge ulcers of missing tissue on every surface. I couldn't see the opening to his windpipe at all and it was clear that it was his own swollen tissues that were blocking his airway. He was running out of time and so was I.

I shaved his leg and gave him an anaesthetic injection because I had to get control of his airway before the entrance disappeared for good. As he slumped onto his side and the gasping stopped I once again showed his owner how to be my nurse and hold his head in the right position for placing a tube into his airway. I couldn't see anything though the swollen tissues, even with the help of a laryngoscope, so I had to rely on years of experience of tubing cats for operations and simply feel my way through the folds. His tongue and mouth had already started to turn blue where he was being starved of oxygen, but after a few short moments I felt the tube slide over the knobbly cartilage of the opening to the airway and the effect was instant and obvious. As I hooked up the tube to the oxygen his breathing eased and his colour returned to pink. It was a relief for now but he was by no means out of the woods. The damage to his mouth and to the back of his throat was substantial and I had no idea whether his brain had been damaged by lack of oxygen. One thing was certain – if I hadn't still been at the surgery by that fluke of timing he never would have made it and I couldn't believe how lucky he had been.

His owner was still pretty shaken, and crying, so I told her to leave him to me and go and sit down and try to calm herself, while I got a better look at what had happened. I gave the cat, whose name I had since found out was Ronan (his owner was later quick to point out that it was after Ronan O'Gara, the rugby player, and not Ronan Keating!), some potent steroids to try to reduce the swelling and inflammation in his mouth, some antibiotics to help combat the bacteria which would have easy access to the bloodstream through all the damaged tissue, and some pain relief because, if he made it out of this, his mouth was going to be hellishly sore.

Once he was stable I got some intravenous fluids started and topped up his anaesthetic so that I could keep him tubed while the swelling started to subside. I called his owner back into the prep room and explained what I thought might have happened. She said there was nothing that she could think of that he might have got hold of at home but he was a very outdoors cat and she had found him in his collapsed state outside the cat flap. The reality was we would probably never know what he'd found and that wasn't going to change anything now anyway. I told her to go home and I would ring her as soon as anything changed for better or worse.

I ended up keeping him totally unconscious for over an hour before I tried the first time to see if he could breathe on his own. It was a disaster. As soon as his reflexes returned and I took the tube out, his throat closed over and I had to start all over again. Eventually it took two more tries and another three hours of anaesthetic to get him conscious and breathing on his own. While he'd been asleep I'd managed to get a good look round his mouth and it was one of the worst sights I'd seen since qualifying. The rough, spiky covering of his tongue was largely missing except for a small strip down the centre. The sides of his tongue were red raw and there were large patches of his cheeks and the back of his throat which looked the same. I had serious doubts about whether he would be able to drink, let alone eat, when he came round and wondered if we were going to need to put a feeding tube into his stomach for days or even weeks while we waited for his mouth to heal.

If there is one thing I've learned over the time I've been qualified, it is that animals are totally and utterly amazing. They have no social hang-ups about disability, they do not complain unless there is something wrong and they have an almost awesome power to get on with the business of living and healing themselves. That very night, after hours of anaesthetic and with a cocktail of drugs on board, Ronan lapped at some special, liquid food I offered. He seemed very hungry and it was clear that it was uncomfortable for him but he managed and I decided to hold off on a stomach tube for now. It had been an intense day by any standards and it was a great phone call to make to let his doting 'mum' know that he seemed to be functioning well and coping with his injuries admirably. He'd pretty much died and been brought back to life about three times but they say cats have nine lives; it seemed he still had some in the bank. Unbelievably, he went home after two days, eating our special food and taking his antibiotics mixed into it. It did take weeks for his mouth to fully heal but outwardly you never would have known. He was a complete star.

Ronan was another one of those cases which was a true emergency, and in my last months in Cheltenham I was destined to see one more dire situation before I could pack myself off up north.

It's a sad fact of veterinary medicine that you get spells which seem to be all doom and gloom, death and sadness. Just as we had all our foreign bodies at once, we seem to get weeks where we suddenly end up having to put lots of animals to sleep for one reason or another. We'd had a run like that not long after I'd seen Ronan and my elation at his recovery had been flattened by the cumulative sadness of what felt like countless owners and the fact that, after years of knowing an animal, it can be very hard for a vet to say goodbye too.

And so it was with a dreadful feeling of foreboding that I waited at the end of morning surgery one day for a lovely couple I knew to bring their little, elderly Jack Russell in. She had apparently collapsed and couldn't walk. I'd known them a while and the dog, Pip, was a real delight to have in but at fifteen she was getting on, even for a terrier. Worst of all they had said on the phone that she had suddenly gone off her front legs, not the usual back ones. This made it much more likely that she had some sort of high spinal or brain disease, which had a much worse outlook than the arthritic changes that usually weaken the back end. I really didn't want to have to tell them that the time had come to say goodbye.

When they arrived I called them straight through and Mr Beaumont was carrying Pip carefully in his arms, cradled protectively to his chest. I gave the couple a sad smile and asked them to tell me exactly what had happened. She'd been absolutely fine and was a very fit dog for her age, as I well knew, and that morning she'd been her normal self. They'd been out for a long walk and after a brief rest at home she'd asked to go in the garden for a sniff about. Literally a few minutes later, they'd looked out to see her falling and staggering round outside, totally unable to use her front legs. They'd rushed her straight down to the practice.

Her little face was poking out of Mr Beaumont's arms, her tongue was lolling, and she was as bright-eyed as ever. It's heartbreaking to have to euthanise animals which are fine and healthy apart from losing the ability to walk. I asked him to put Pip on the floor so that I could see for myself exactly how she moved and the extent of the disability. Sure enough, as soon as she hit the floor she fell sideways, with her front feet unable to move and scrabbling with her back legs to maintain balance, but she just couldn't manage. She tumbled this way and that as she tried with all her might to compensate for whatever it was that had befallen her. It really was quite shocking to see, and her owners' faces were a picture of worry. After a few moments of watching her, there was one thing that really caught my eye and a tiny glimmer of hope started to surface but I couldn't really believe what I thought I was seeing. She looked like she couldn't actually separate her front feet for some reason. I squatted down and peered closer, and a frown started to wrinkle my brow as I hoped with all my might I was right. I caught hold of her by the shoulders and gently pulled her towards me. Her two front dewclaws were quite long and had become snagged together like a little pair of home-made handcuffs. It seemed too bizarre to be true, but, as I unhooked them from each other and let her go, she stood, gave herself a good shake, started furiously wagging her tail and trotted, totally normally, to the door of the consulting room. She stood there, looking over her shoulder at her owners with an expression that quite clearly said she thought it was time to go now.

I couldn't stop the huge beaming smile that was appearing on my face and it soon turned into an uncontrollable giggle as Mr and Mrs Beaumont looked at me disbelievingly and then both simultaneously went scarlet with embarrassment. They both started apologising profusely for wasting my time and kept saying they just couldn't believe that was all it was. For my part I was laughing so much I couldn't really speak and just shook my head happily and told them I was over the moon because we'd had such a sad run recently. I couldn't have been happier. Mr Beaumont was reaching for his wallet and asking how much they owed but I shook my head and sent them home because this was one occasion where money really wasn't needed, not when the outcome was so priceless.

I told Mark about it on the phone that evening and was chuckling away about the rarity of such a thing when he told me he'd had a similar emergency himself once. He had just seen the last client of the evening and was finishing up the records when one of the nurses came in and said they had one more client on the way with an emergency that they had had to tell to come straight down. The woman sounded on the verge of tears and the nurse told Mark that apparently the woman had said her cat's 'guts were all hanging out'.

Obviously this sounded very serious and between them Mark and the nurse had started getting together all the things they might conceivably need to get the cat's treatment started and they began to get the operating theatre ready too.

After busying themselves doing all that, there was only a couple of minutes to wait before the woman rushed through the door with her little ginger cat crouched in his basket, wide-eyed and bewildered at his sudden change of surroundings. Mark took them straight in and gently lifted the cat out as he started asking the owner what had happened. There didn't seem to be a huge mass of intestine immediately obvious, so Mark gently laid the cat over onto his side as the woman pointed and breathlessly said, 'Look. There!'

'Do you mean this?' Mark replied as he gingerly picked a large garden slug from the cat's coat. Of course the woman was mortally embarrassed but Mark thought it was brilliant and, again, no payment required!

My last week at the practice was an odd mix of sadness at leaving all the friends, clients and animals I'd met in my seven years in the area and the excitement of moving on to new things and the fact that finally Mark and I would be together all the time. Alison threw a lovely get-together for me, inviting the clients she knew I was closest to, and she'd made me a montage of photos of my time there. I apologised once again for leaving her after she'd been so good to me but she just smiled, said, 'Just make sure I get an invite to the wedding,' and winked.

In my last evening surgery my very last clients of the day, and therefore of my time in Cheltenham, were a great couple I knew well who had a pair of Dalmatians. One of the dogs had been in for a vaccination and we were chewing the fat afterwards because I knew I didn't have anyone else to see. The computer was idling away just behind me and I gradually became aware that the man of the duo, Bill, was staring intently and slightly frowning. I lost the stream of what I was saying and started looking at him. He turned to me and said, 'Does that say what I think it does?'

I turned to see what he was referring to and it took me a couple of seconds to see what was different about our screen saver, which usually bounced slowly round the screen showing the name of the practice, 'Vets on the Park'. Somehow now the words 'Vets in the Dark' were making their leisurely way round the screen. I started smiling and looked to where Julie was standing in the doorway. As our gaze met she quickly averted her eyes and walked away into the waiting room, nonchalantly whistling as she went, and with a smile on her face. I suppose as a parting shot it could have been worse. She told me afterwards over our goodbye glass of wine that she had planned to change it to 'Vets on the Piss' but had bottled out at the last minute!

Although we were pretty sure of how we felt about each other and I couldn't wait to make the move, there was also a part of me that was scared at the same time. By the very nature of the fact that I was making another huge change in my life, it was clear that by the age of thirty-three I still hadn't had a relationship which had worked. While my heart said, 'go, go, go', my head said, 'go, but don't sell your house just yet in case you need to come back!' This was advice echoed by my parents, who were still looking out for their 'little girl' and were quite clearly worried about my impetuous decision. I couldn't blame them. From the outside I'm sure it looked like I was throwing away the first job I'd really loved and leaving all my friends and stability behind because of what amounted to a holiday romance. I hoped this time they wouldn't be as annoyingly right as parents usually turn out to be.

The actual move itself happened pretty gradually over a number of weeks. Mark and I had been spending weekends racing back and forth between York and Cheltenham to spend as much time as possible together. This had become fairly one-sided for a couple of months because Mark had ruptured his Achilles tendon (which he was very upset to learn from the Internet is an injury most commonly seen in 'middle-aged men') playing basketball, and had therefore had to resort to the train, or have me do all the driving. As it had transpired, Mark had been in the process of moving house himself when we'd met and his injury had delayed the exchange of contracts. When he finally moved that September it had coincided with me handing in my notice, so I had ended up with three months to gradually take my belongings north every time I went visiting. At the beginning of December we hired a van and heaved the last of the furniture in, obviously taking care not to strain any more of Mark's middle-aged bits! With the cats and dogs in the car, with the house up for rent, and bursting with excitement and anticipation, we set off in convoy to start the next chapter in my life.

The house Mark had bought, and that my animals and I moved into, was in a beautiful little village. Having moved fairly often before, all the animals soon adjusted admirably and made themselves well and truly at home. The people who'd lived in the house before us had no pets, so one of our first jobs was fitting a cat flap. Now, without laying blame at anyone's door, there was a slight mix-up with the measurements and we ended up having to make a trip back to the pet shop to get a bigger cat flap because the one we'd bought just fell straight through the enormous hole we'd made. It was clear already that surgery tools obviously sat more comfortably with both of us than woodworking ones. One night, soon after the medium-sized flap had been successfully installed (and after some joking from friends that if we carried on the way we were going we'd end up with a burglar flap), I woke with a start in the middle of the night to some very eerie howling, which sounded exactly like a wolf. It was clearly coming from just outside the house so I raced downstairs to find Pan sitting looking very melancholy indeed outside the back door. It was three o'clock in the morning and freezing cold. I felt dreadful. I must have accidentally shut him out when the boys went out for their night-time wee. What a terrible mother I was.

The next night I let the boys in from their pre-bedtime foray, shut and locked the back door and gave them their treats. Then, for the sake of my own sanity, I asked Mark to bear witness to the fact that both dogs were well and truly inside the house. Sure enough, at about four o'clock I once again woke to howling and found Pan in the back garden. We were totally flummoxed. I went round testing all the doors and finally came to the conclusion that he must be getting out the cat flap. Now I know I said it was a big flap but this was still not an easy conclusion to draw. Our dogs are about the size of tall Labradors and weigh 30 kilos apiece. Later that day I got to see, or hear, first-hand that this was exactly what was going on. I was working at the computer and heard an almighty clattering and got into the hallway just in time to see Pan's tail disappearing out the flap into the garden. I went outside and saw him straining and realised the upset tummy he'd had for a couple of days was obviously making him desperate enough to wedge himself through the small hole in the night rather than soil the house. It was still difficult to imagine so, when he'd finished, I put him indoors and then told him to go out through the flap and watched in amazement as he seemed to elongate his body and somehow get through. This was when I discovered that the build of the plastic flap didn't allow the door to fully open the other way, which was why every time he went out he got stuck the other side. I had to admire both his cleanliness and his ingenuity, and I hoped the neighbours had more soundproof windows than we did and hadn't heard him howling the last two nights.

Quite fortunately for the animals, the cats that Mark had had when he'd been married some years before now lived a couple of miles away with his ex-wife (although he still saw to their veterinary needs). This meant that my motley crew didn't have to get used to any foreign animals on their new patch. I needn't have worried about the effect the upheaval might have, though, because before long it became quite clear just how at home they all were.

A few months after we had moved in, the window cleaners had been and I was at the door sorting out the money when one of them said, 'Erm, have you got cats?'

'Yes, we've got three, why?'

'Well, er, there's a big dead hamster in your back garden.'

I wasn't really sure what to say to this and assured him that I would look into it. I thought he must just be mistaken and that he'd seen a dead vole or mouse or something and mistaken it for a hamster. I wandered out into the garden and, to my horror, there in the middle of the lawn was a huge, black, pet hamster, stiff as a board and quite dead. I found myself glancing shiftily around, like a murderer caught in the act, and muttered a single word under my breath as I picked the stiff creature up by the smallest tip of a foot that I could and headed for the dustbin. Brian.

Living in a small village, and having learnt my lesson with the near-fatal budgie incident in Cheltenham, and knowing that everyone here knew that the new couple on the block were both vets, I decided that my best course of action was to maintain a guilty silence. So the hamster went unmentioned and we never heard anyone enquiring about a missing pet, so maybe it had been a wild hamster. In North Yorkshire? I'm sure stranger things have happened.

Brian was obviously feeling like he was getting the lie of the land and, in our own foraging expeditions, Mark and I had found a great local pub which, most importantly, was dog friendly. We started to go a couple of times a week and quickly felt very welcomed by Maria and Andrew, the landlady and landlord, and by the locals. Pan, of course, loved it because they had a dartboard. After a short while he was so well known in there that, if he was sitting faithfully under the board waiting for a game, there was always someone who would have one just for him. It got to the stage that the dogs would get more excited at the thought of going to the pub than just about anything else and, when they thought that's where we were heading, it was the only time they would scrabble and whine to get out of the house.

One night we were going out into town for dinner with our neighbours, Ian and Margaret, who we'd got to know and still love spending time with. We'd decided to have a glass of wine at their house first, before the taxi came, and the boys came with us as they always did. When it was time to go we opened our own door, ushered the dogs inside, locked up, jumped in the taxi and headed off for a lovely meal and a relaxing night. When we got home a couple of hours later we found a note on the front door which said, 'Dogs at the pub, all fine, come round when you're back.'

This was bewildering so we trooped off round the corner and found that Pan and Badger were very happy indeed nestled in the cottage next door to the pub with Andrew and Maria, the pub itself now being closed. But what on earth had happened? Well, it transpired that Andrew had been behind the bar and had seen Badger wander in the open door and assumed we would appear behind him any minute. Sometime later there was no sign of us and by this time Badger was sitting with a family who were having their dinner in there and was very happily taking the numerous chips they were offering. Andrew assumed he must have been mistaken and that the dog wasn't

Badger but belonged to the family. When they'd finished and were about to leave they went to the bar and asked Andrew if it was OK to give the dog the remains of their pie crust. Apparently he'd thought to himself, 'Well, it's your dog, you can do what you like', so told them of course they could. It wasn't until five minutes after they'd gone that he realised that Badger was still there and that the family must have thought he was a pub dog. He'd called Badger and wandered round to our house with him to find no one home and Pan stuck in the back garden, sitting by the back gate looking very miserable and lonely. He'd then released Pan from his garden prison, taken both dogs back with him, and come back to leave the note. It's one of those times that every pet owner has had where you wish you could see a video of what happened. We can only surmise that the boys had been very excited at the thought of going to the pub and had then thought when we put them back in the house, that we'd gone to the pub without them. This was clearly unforgiveable so they'd immediately legged it out the cat flap, whereupon Badger had managed to find a hole in the fence and go to the pub, but Pan, the more headless chicken of the two, hadn't. He had just sat at the gate and waited. I suppose that I should be embarrassed or even slightly ashamed that our dogs are so habituated to the pub that they actually *went on their own without us* but I can't help feeling just a little bit proud of them too.

The animals, it seemed, had found their niche, and, after a few months of dossing around the house, it was time for me to do so too because there finally arose an opportunity at Mark's practice for me to start working there. I'd moved north without a job to go to and, for the first time in my life, had had to get used to being a 'kept woman'. Having been brought up most definitely to pay my way it had been difficult to adjust to at first, and, after several months of having a wonderfully lazy time, I was ready to get my hands dirty again. Working at Mark's practice was perfect because it's a huge place so we could work together virtually without ever seeing each other. I'd never worked somewhere that size and found I really enjoyed it. They still had a big emphasis on continuity by having lots of smaller branches, which really appealed to me, but suddenly, almost ten years after graduating, I was surrounded by lots of vets, nurses, kennel maids and receptionists, and working in yet another very different environment.

It was great to start again and meet new clients and their animals, and also to start forging work relationships. Mark's practice was very young at heart and I found the vets great fun to work, and socialise with, and soon enough we were exchanging stories. You always think you've seen the weirdest things or met the maddest people or had the biggest nightmare, but it's important to talk because there'll always be someone worse off than you and in this case it was the locum I would be replacing. Tom was a very good-looking young Australian vet, who'd come to England to get a bit of experience and see the world. He'd had a great few months and was torn about whether to stay but eventually family had won out and he'd decided to go back to the sunny side of the world. At his farewell do he'd told me, with a twinkle in his eye, about two of his most memorable moments working for the practice.

He'd been brought a small puppy to vaccinate, nothing too taxing, and had launched into his well-rehearsed patter about everything that an enthusiastic new puppy owner needs to know. After a few moments of chatting he grabbed his stethoscope and started his clinical examination of the very cute and very wriggly little cocker spaniel. The puppy was trying desperately to leap about and lick his face, so the rather, shall we say, curvaceous owner had to hold the puppy firmly to her chest. Tom had already listened to one side of the puppy's chest but, being thorough, and being on autopilot, he'd reached his hand firmly round to listen to the other side of the heart and lungs. It took about two seconds for him to realise that he had plunged his hand inside the woman's low-cut top and that his hand was wedged right between her warm bosoms. He'd whipped his hand out and got very flustered, apologised and rattled through the rest of the consultation without giving her a single second to say anything. Afterwards, he'd spent a day or two fretting about getting sued for all sorts of lewd behaviour, so he'd gone to talk to one of the partners about what had happened. He'd advised him to ring the VDS (Veterinary Defence Society) to get some advice and to give them a heads-up that they might have a complaint coming. They made a note of everything that had happened but told him they'd received no complaint as yet. Only time would tell. About a couple of weeks later he saw the woman and the puppy back on his list and broke into a cold sweat. He went to see the receptionist who'd booked it in and told her she had to change it to another vet because he simply couldn't see her again. This was when he found out that she had specifically asked for him and most definitely didn't want to see anyone else! Apparently it had been the longest ten minutes of his life while he tried steadfastly to ignore the fact that she was done up to the nines, smothered in perfume and had an even lower cut to her neckline that day. This time he made sure a nurse was in there to help him hold the puppy for its second vaccination.

It seemed he had only just about recovered from the trauma of this encounter when he was on duty one night and was called out to a cat that was bleeding profusely from its mouth. He met the couple, both female, at the surgery and quickly ascertained that the blood was coming from a tooth, which had broken off well below the gum line. The cat was being very amiable so he told them the best thing he could do was simply apply some pressure to the site until the bleeding stopped. After a couple of minutes he took his thumb away and the blood stubbornly started again as if he had done nothing. Being a bright and optimistic sort he was unshaken, told them not to worry and said that all he needed to do was give it a bit longer and this time he would wait exactly five minutes before he let go. That should definitely do the job. Five minutes is actually quite a long time to stand and do nothing and soon enough the polite conversation dried up and an awkward silence settled over the room. He smiled at the pair and looked away, desperately trying to think of something to say. Eventually his face brightened as the perfect analogy popped into his head and he blurted it out before his brain had a chance to intervene and shout at him to keep his mouth shut.

'Ha ha,' he said, 'I feel just like that little Dutch boy with his finger in the dyke.' The stony silence that ensued made the earlier awkward silence seem like a party.

I'd been worried that having several months off after moving to Yorkshire might have made me forget everything I'd ever been taught, but he made me smile with his stories, and I realised that everything would be all right. Soon enough I was settled once again into the routine and the ups and downs of general practice.

I've come to realise over the years that having a veterinary degree really is a ticket to anywhere and that there are so many things you can do with it. Since meeting Mark I've got involved with student teaching, numerous animal welfare charities and the British Veterinary Association, and I have become very involved in welfare matters like tail docking and pedigree breeding. I've met and worked alongside a huge number of inspiring vets who, just like Alison, have restored my faith in my initial passion to be a vet, to be part of a brilliant and caring profession.

When I was seeing practice while I was still at school, before I even had a place at vet school, I was desperate to be a vet. But some of the vets that I saw practice with confided in me that they never told anyone they were vets if they were out socially with people who didn't know. They would never admit at a party that that was their job and some had fantastic fabricated careers to divert people away from the truth. I was always stunned when, as a wide-eyed and naive sixteen-year-old, I heard this. Wow, I thought, if I ever get to be a vet I'm going to shout it from the rooftops. I'll be the proudest vet in the world. But they would say to me that if you tell people you're a vet they will talk about nothing else. Your whole world starts to revolve around it and the fact is, they would say, that there are some times that you just don't want to be that professional pillar of the community and talk about other people's animals after a long day, week or month of talking about other people's animals. This seemed inconceivable to me but the years in the job have made me see their point to a degree. There are indeed times that it would be nice to be anonymous, to be silly, to shed the serious and often sombre mask of an everyday vet. The television career I've had made this impossible for me because millions of people already know I'm a vet before I have a chance to lie about it but I've also seen that 'normal' vets can struggle to hide too.

A few years after meeting, Mark and I decided to get married and, as many men do, he went off for a stag weekend, organised by one of his three (he clearly can't make decisions) best men. Birmingham was picked for reasons best known to Richard, the man in question, but probably because it was near his home turf, making the organisation much easier. For Mark there would be no worries about letting his hair down and being caught doing something silly in front of an unsuspecting client. But Richard had clearly not thought about the consequences of being on his own patch.

A 'few beers' had been consumed and the party had inevitably ended up in the type of place where ladies do their best to entertain the inebriated masses by dancing in a provocative, yet sophisticated, way. In other words, they went to a strip club. All was going well, Mark was being suitably humiliated for everyone to see and was trying his best to fade into the background when he was saved by a beautiful, young, scantily clad woman. She walked straight up to Richard, in front of everyone, and beamed her gorgeous smile at him. 'Oh, it's you,' she gushed, clearly in awe of him for some reason.

The others looked on with an amused and sudden interest in what they thought might turn out to be some very juicy gossip to take back to his partner, who they all knew very well would kill him if he'd been in the slightest bit bad. Richard was looking a bit confused and embarrassed and it was clear he couldn't quite remember through the beer haze how he knew this lovely lady. She turned to the assembled masses, put her arm round him and leaned against him in a big squeeze of a hug, balancing the tray of beers she was carrying precariously in one hand. She finally released him and gave him a drink on the house before telling everyone he was a wonderful vet and looked after her numerous guinea pigs better than anyone had ever done. Mark may have been the one who came back with the whip bruises on his buttocks but, by the sound of it, Richard was the one who was most deeply embarrassed that night.

The veterinary world is a small one and you often find you bump into the same people time and again. After a few years of being up north I'd made lots of great veterinary acquaintances, whom I'd catch up with once or twice a year when we happened to end up thrown together on some course or another. One summer Mark and I had booked onto a weekend of learning combined with various sporting options. There would be lectures morning and evening and a variety of activities during the afternoon. On the Saturday I had stupidly agreed to go mountain biking with a group of the vets, who had assured me it would be a gentle outing with maybe a pub lunch followed by a slow amble back in plenty of time for a shower before lectures that evening.

Twenty-six miles later I was cursing everyone and my own stupidity and was on the verge of a tantrum and physical collapse. We returned with about two minutes to spare before we had to run to lectures caked in sweat, mud and, in my case, tears from when I had thrown my toys out of the pram when I'd seen the last 'gentle' hill we'd had to climb. Needless to say, all this physical activity had given all of us quite a thirst and a need to unwind. The course was being held in a lovely country hotel in the Peak District and that night we'd dug ourselves in at the bar and were having a lovely time. There was a wedding reception going on elsewhere, with guests spilling over into the bar, and then a hen party arrived. Our motley crew had taken up residence on some big settees in one corner and the hen party, complete with the hen's grandma, took the seats opposite us. A few pleasantries had been exchanged across a very crowded and noisy bar and, as the night went on, one particularly entertaining soul from our party had thought he would give the hen party a treat by doing a very unforgettable rendition of Alice Cooper's 'Poison', which so clearly traumatised the hen's grandmother that we had to reel him back over to our side and sit on him until the jukebox finally started playing a song he didn't know.

I don't know if it's a trait particular to vets or simply to any group of men, some of whom in this instance were from the Welsh valleys, but soon enough there were quite a few men in the group singing in a robust way about anything from country roads in West Virginia to Ilkley Moor and everyone was having a very relaxing end to a tiring day. One of our party, Steve, took the floor and started a powerful and brilliantly heartfelt rendition of 'Swing Low, Sweet Chariot'. This turned out to involve a couple of rounds of singing with the actions and then rounds where the words became fewer and fewer until he was standing tall among us. While we looked on in awe, he carried on valiantly doing just the actions and not singing a word.

It was at this point that, bizarrely, from across the room, the hen suddenly stood up, pointed straight at him and shouted, '*That's* where I know you from. You're our vet.' There was a sudden and deathly silence as Steve stood, stock-still, mid imaginary chariot ride, looking for all the world like a slightly pallid and scrawny Ben Hur, and cast his eyes sideways to where the whole hen party was staring at him. We were only just starting to realise the wonderful mileage in this when one of her relatives piped up with the brilliantly damning, 'Ooh, yes, that's right. You killed our dog, Frankie. You ruined our Christmas!'

Steve's arms dropped listlessly to his side as the air was taken clean out of him. He straightened up, bowed his head, assumed a very sombre air and apologetically sat down, while the rest of us wept mercilessly with laughter at his expense. So you see, this is my plea to you. Whatever your views on us vets are, good or bad, I ask you to remember this; we're only human and, no matter what we have to do in our line of work, there are still some things that really shouldn't happen to a vet.

Afterword

So that's the recipe for this vet's life and now you might be wondering if it's time to stick a fork in me and turn me over to see if I'm done. The answer, as always in life, is 'Who knows?' But I can tell you three things of which I'm sure:

- So far, my relationship track record seems to be improving and Mark still hasn't realised he's way out of my league.

- I'm still as passionate about animals and their welfare as I ever was, and I will continue striving to make a difference however I can.

- As for the hands-on, dirty business of being involved with the tail end of our planet's wonderful animals, well, that is on hold for now. Don't worry, though, I still spend every day immersed in what feels like a sea of poo and various bodily fluids. It seems that the two beautiful daughters Mark and I have produced have helped me to succeed in something I never thought possible: apparently a vet can, after repeated exposure, finally get used to the grossest species I've come across – humans!

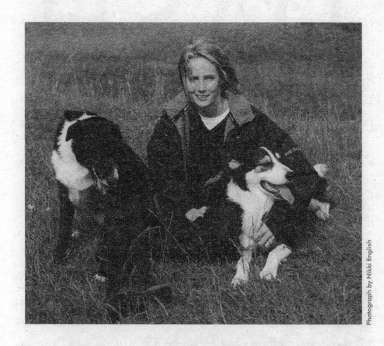

Photograph by Nikki English

This book is dedicated to the memory of Pan and Badger.
You were the most wonderful dogs in the world and my best
friends for fifteen years. I love you, boys.

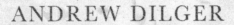

ANDREW DILGER

DASH

Bitch of the Year

Champion racer
to ring bearer...
in twelve
months flat

*'I fell in love with Dash in this
thoroughly enjoyable book...
It's funny, moving and
I highly recommend it'*

TWIGGY

DASH
Bitch of the Year

ISBN: 978-1-84953-118-4   Paperback   £7.99

'Bed.' I patted it. 'Bed.' We both looked at the bed like schoolkids staring at the Rosetta Stone. I crouched down and curled up in the bed, with my legs hanging out and my head over the side. Dash gave an enormous yawn, as if wanting to know what on earth I was doing. I asked myself the same question. It was going to be a long afternoon.

Andrew had always wanted a dog – something you could mould into the perfect playmate. Tail going like a windscreen wiper, tongue a pink strip, wet-nosed, bright-eyed – what boy wouldn't want such a force in his life? But a man of thirty-seven, just about to propose to his girlfriend? And an ex-racing greyhound?

Dash is a heart-warming memoir about the adoption of a champion greyhound and her transformation into ring bearer at her new owner's wedding. 'Dash' is far from perfect, but that's half the fun. The novelty of a man trying to organise a wedding is the other half.

'a must for all dog lovers, everyone contemplating dog ownership and everyone contemplating marriage.'   Barbara Erskine

'heart-warming'   OXFORDSHIRE LIMITED EDITION

'an endearing, amusing tale that will resonate with dog-lovers – and romantics – everywhere.'   THE GOOD BOOK GUIDE

Twenty Wagging Tales

Our Year of Rehoming Orphan Dogs

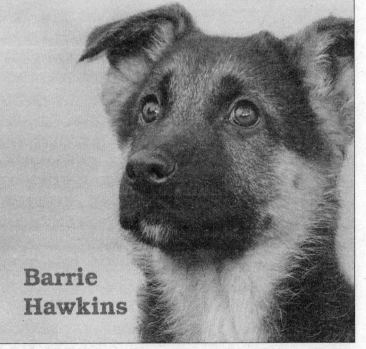

Barrie
Hawkins

TWENTY WAGGING TALES
Our Year of Rehoming Orphan Dogs

ISBN: 978-1-84024-755-8   Paperback   £8.99

'*What a day! A dog from a car-breaker's yard on the loose with no lead and not even a collar, bathing a guard dog who had known me for an hour and trying to towel him in a room hardly any bigger than a cupboard, dirty water shaken all over me...*'

This heart-warming and often hilarious tale follows a year in the life of Barrie and Dorothy Hawkins, who don't quite realise what they are letting themselves in for when they take on the challenge of rescuing and rehoming orphan dogs.

It seems every canine character has a surprise in store: Monty, the dog with a taste for cheese; Oscar, who has never been played with or walked but develops a new zest for life at the age of twelve; Digby, the enormous ex-guard dog who when he's not squashing the daisies is squashing Barrie's foot...

The husband and wife team welcome them all into their hearts and do everything it takes to change their lives for the better – and the lives of their new owners, too.

'*a chatty and engaging memoir, packed with amusing anecdotes.*'
CAMBRIDGESHIRE JOURNAL

'*good-natured story-telling, judicious use of self-deprecating humor and a genuine love of its subject.*'
WASHINGTON POST

Have you enjoyed this book?
If so, why not write a review on your favourite website?

Thanks very much for buying this Summersdale book.

www.summersdale.com